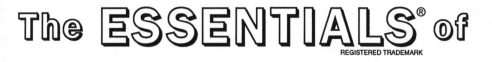

The ESSENTIALS® of

REGISTERED TRADEMARK

BIOCHEMISTRY

Jay M. Templin, Ed.D.

Professor, Biology Department
College of New Jersey
Trenton, New Jersey

D0197642

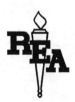

Research and Education Association
61 Ethel Road West
Piscataway, New Jersey 08854

THE ESSENTIALS ®
OF BIOCHEMISTRY

1998 PRINTING

Printed in the United States of America

Library of Congress Catalog Card Number 97-65224

International Standard Book Number 0-87891-073-5

WHAT "THE ESSENTIALS" WILL DO FOR YOU

This book is a review and study guide. It is comprehensive and it is concise.

It helps in preparing for exams, in doing homework, and remains a handy reference source at all times.

It condenses the vast amount of detail characteristic of the subject matter and summarizes the **essentials** of the field.

It will thus save hours of study and preparation time.

The book provides quick access to the important principles, pathways, structures, and functions in the field.

Materials needed for exams can be reviewed in summary form – eliminating the need to read and reread many pages of textbook and class notes. The summaries will even tend to bring detail to mind that had been previously read or noted.

This "ESSENTIALS" book has been prepared by an expert in the field, and has been carefully reviewed to assure accuracy and maximum usefulness.

Dr. Max Fogiel
Program Director

CONTENTS

Chapter 3
BIOENERGETICS AND CELL STRUCTURE

Chapter 4
CARBOHYDRATES—STRUCTURE AND FUNCTION

Chapter 5
LIPIDS—STRUCTURE AND FUNCTION

Chapter 6
PROTEIN DIGESTION AND METABOLISM

Chapter 7
NUCLEIC ACIDS—STRUCTURE AND FUNCTION

Chapter 8
EXTRACELLULAR FLUID/HOMEOSTASIS

Chapter 9
GLOSSARY OF TERMS 72

THE PERIODIC TABLE

METALS **NONMETALS**

KEY
112.40	← Atomic weight
Cd	← Symbol
48	← Atomic number

TRANSITION METALS

PERIODS	IA	IIA	IIIB	IVB	VB	VIB	VIIB	VIII			IB	IIB	IIIA	IVA	VA	VIA	VIIA	O
1	1.0079 H 1																1.0079 H 1	4.00260 He 2
2	6.94 Li 3	9.01218 Be 4											10.81 B 5	12.011 C 6	14.0067 N 7	15.9994 O 8	18.9984 F 9	20.179 Ne 10
3	22.9898 Na 11	24.305 Mg 12											26.9815 Al 13	28.086 Si 14	30.9738 P 15	32.06 S 16	35.453 Cl 17	39.948 Ar 18
4	39.098 K 19	40.08 Ca 20	44.9559 Sc 21	47.90 Ti 22	50.9414 V 23	51.996 Cr 24	54.9380 Mn 25	55.847 Fe 26	58.9332 Co 27	58.71 Ni 28	63.546 Cu 29	65.38 Zn 30	69.72 Ga 31	72.59 Ge 32	74.9216 As 33	78.96 Se 34	79.904 Br 35	83.80 Kr 36
5	85.4678 Rb 37	87.62 Sr 38	88.9059 Y 39	91.22 Zr 40	92.9064 Nb 41	95.94 Mo 42	98.9062 Tc 43	101.07 Ru 44	102.9055 Rh 45	106.4 Pd 46	107.868 Ag 47	112.40 Cd 48	114.82 In 49	118.69 Sn 50	121.75 Sb 51	127.60 Te 52	126.9046 I 53	131.30 Xe 54
6	132.9054 Cs 55	137.34 Ba 56	57–71 *	178.49 Hf 72	180.9479 Ta 73	183.85 W 74	186.2 Re 75	190.2 Os 76	192.22 Ir 77	195.09 Pt 78	196.9665 Au 79	200.59 Hg 80	204.37 Tl 81	207.2 Pb 82	208.9804 Bi 83	(210) Po 84	(210) At 85	(222) Rn 86
7	(223) Fr 87	(226.0254) Ra 88	89–103 †	(260) Ku 104	(260) Ha 105													

* LANTHANIDE SERIES

138.9055 La 57	140.12 Ce 58	140.9077 Pr 59	144.24 Nd 60	(145) Pm 61	150.4 Sm 62	151.96 Eu 63	157.25 Gd 64	158.9254 Tb 65	162.50 Dy 66	164.9304 Ho 67	167.26 Er 68	168.9342 Tm 69	173.04 Yb 70	174.97 Lu 71

† ACTINIDE SERIES

(227) Ac 89	232.0381 Th 90	231.0359 Pa 91	238.029 U 92	237.0482 Np 93	(242) Pu 94	(243) Am 95	(245) Cm 96	(245) Bk 97	(248) Cf 98	(253) Es 99	(254) Fm 100	(256) Md 101	(253) No 102	(257) Lr 103

CHAPTER 1

Biological Structure/ Chemistry of Proteins

1.1 Introduction to Biochemistry

1.1.1 What is Biochemistry?

Chemistry is the study of the structure of matter. Matter is anything that has mass and volume. **Biochemistry** focuses specifically on the **molecules** of matter, **biomolecules**, composing living organisms. There are four main classes of important biomolecules: **proteins, carbohydrates, lipids,** and **nucleic acids.**

Biochemistry also relates the structure to the function of biomolecules. **Starch,** for example, is a complex carbohydrate, or **polysaccharide**. This large molecule consists of many smaller subunits—**glucose** molecules—which are **monosaccharides**. When starch is consumed, it is chemically digested into smaller glucose molecules. Glucose, or blood sugar, serves as a source of energy for the estimated 100 trillion cells of the human body.

A knowledge of biochemistry provides an important foundation for understanding all fields of the life sciences, including **microbiology** and **genetics**. For example, some antibiotics work by disrupting the protein synthesis machinery of a disease-causing bacterium. **DNA** is a **nucleic acid** that encodes the genetic information for the development of an organism's traits, such as eye color and blood type.

1.1.2 Fields of Biochemistry

The answers to many questions in biology are found at the molecular level. Therefore, other fields that draw on biochemistry include **cell biology, zoology, botany, anatomy, physiology,** and **ecology.**

1.2 Polymers/Subunits/Functional Groups

1.2.1 Structure of Polymers

Although many biomolecules are large and complex, they consist of simpler molecules that are bonded together. These smaller molecules are **subunits,** or building blocks. **RNA,** for example, is a nucleic acid. This long, chain-like molecule consists of four kinds of simpler subunits, **nucleotides,** bonded together in the chain.

A **polymer** is a large molecule consisting of smaller molecules that are bonded together. Among the four classes of biomolecules, examples of polymers and their bonded subunits are as follows:

Classes	*Polymers*	*Subunits*
protein	polypeptide	amino acid
carbohydrate	polysaccharide	monosaccharide
lipid	triglyceride	fatty acid, glycerol
nucleic acid	DNA, RNA	nucleotide

1.2.2 Functional Groups

There are certain **functional groups** that form the structure of polymers and their subunits. These functional groups determine the shape and properties of these polymers. An **enzyme,** for example, is mainly a protein. It must have a specific shape to fit into another molecule and make it reactive. By doing this, an enzyme acts as a **catalyst.** It speeds up the rate of a chemical reaction.

The **structural formulas** for some of the major functional groups in biomolecules are shown in Figure 1–1. A structural formula shows the spatial relationship between **atoms** that are bonded together. **Elements,**

2

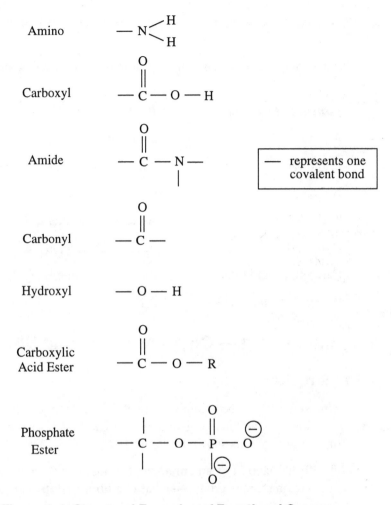

Figure 1–1: Structural Formulas of Functional Groups

the simplest substances, occur as distinct particles called atoms. All of the basic principles of chemistry apply to biochemistry. Note that the four most common elements in biomolecules are **carbon, nitrogen, oxygen,** and **hydrogen.**

Atoms unite to form **molecules** by forming **covalent bonds.** A covalent bond has one pair of electrons that is shared between the outer-

3

most energy shells of two atoms. A carbon atom forms four covalent bonds. Nitrogen forms three bonds, while oxygen forms two and hydrogen forms one.

Some of the major functional groups in biomolecules are as follows:

Functional Groups	*Biomolecules*
Amino	amino acid
Carboxyl	amino acid, fatty acid
Amide	bonds amino acids in proteins
Carbonyl	some monosaccharides
Hydroxyl	monosaccharide, glycerol
Carboxylic acid ester	triglycerides among lipids
Phosphate ester	ATP

1.3 Amino Acids—Characteristics and Structure

1.3.1 Structure

Amino acids are the subunits of **proteins**. Twenty different amino acids commonly occur in living organisms. The general structural formula for an amino acid is shown in Figure 1–2.

The **alpha carbon** of an amino acid forms four covalent bonds. It bonds to two functional groups—a basic **amino group** and an acidic

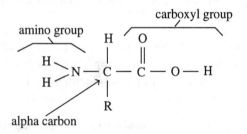

Figure 1–2: Structural Formula of an Amino Acid

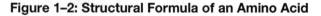

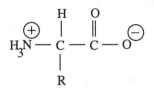

Figure 1–3: Amino Acid as a Zwitterion

---

carboxyl group. A hydrogen atom is also covalently bonded to this carbon. Amino acids share these three bonded groups in common. However, they differ by the identity of a fourth bonded group, the **R group**.

1.3.2 Amino Acids in Water

The R group is different for each amino acid. In the amino acid **glycine**, for example, the R group is a covalently bonded hydrogen atom. In the amino acid **leucine**, the R group includes a long carbon chain. For **tryptophan**, part of the R group is two carbon rings.

The R group of an amino acid can be **hydrophilic** (water-attracting) or **hydrophobic** (water-repelling). When dissolved in water, the arrangement of hydrophilic and hydrophobic R groups of bonded amino acids determines the shape of the protein molecule. Hydrophobic groups attract each other and away from water. Hydrophilic groups are often on the surface of a protein structure and orient toward water.

Unbonded amino acids have **acid-base** properties when dissolved in water. The carboxyl group tends to lose a proton (positive charge) and become negative, a property of **acids**. The amino group tends to accept a proton and become positive, a property of **bases**. Therefore, an amino acid can have a positive and a negative end. This dipolar ion is called a **zwitterion** (see Figure 1–3). Note that the entire amino acid is neutral.

A zwitterion has many properties in common with **salts**, compounds consisting of positive and negative ions (e.g., NaCl). Therefore, unbonded amino acids are crystalline and soluble in water. They also have high melting points.

1.3.3 Amino Acids and pH

In an acidic solution (many protons, with pH less than 7), amino acids accept protons on their negative ends. In basic solutions (fewer protons, with pH higher than 7), they lose protons from their positive ends. The **isoelectric point** is the pH at which the number of positive and negative charges is equal in an amino acid in solution. For example, the isoelectric point for alanine is 6.0.

The isoelectric point influences the charge for each amino acid sample dissolved in water. Amino acids can dissolve in **plasma**, the liquid part of the **blood**. Plasma is mostly water. The pH of human blood is about 7.4. This value is basic and above the isoelectric point for alanine. Therefore, in blood, alanine tends to lose protons and becomes negative.

1.4 Proteins—Chemistry and Structure

1.4.1 Structure

Proteins are polymers of covalently bonded amino acids. Figure 1–4 shows how two amino acids can bond, with the accompanying loss of a water molecule. This union is a **peptide bond**. The larger molecule

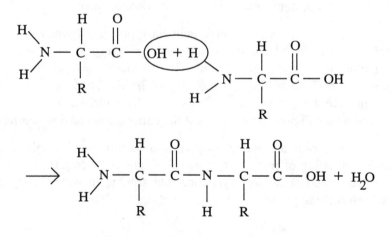

Figure 1–4: Formation of a Dipeptide

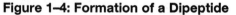

is a **dipeptide**. A **tripeptide** consists of three bonded amino acids. Cells have the ability to make long, chain-like polymers of bonded amino acids. A **polypeptide** consists of 10 to 100 bonded amino acids. A protein is larger.

1.4.2 Levels of Structure

Proteins have four levels of structure.

The **primary structure** is the sequence of amino acids covalently bonded together. With 20 amino acids in cells, the possibilities for different sequences are endless.

The primary structure determines the other levels of structure and the overall shape of the protein molecule. In sickle cell anemia, a change in only 1 of the 146 amino acids in a polypeptide of **hemoglobin** changes the properties of this molecule. Located in human **erythrocytes** (red blood cells), the hemoglobin molecule normally transports oxygen. Sickle cell hemoglobin loses this ability.

Secondary structure is the result of the amino acid sequence of the polypeptide. It represents the most stable form for the conditions encountered by the polypeptide. Hydrogen bonding between amino acids of the polypeptide is responsible for the stability of secondary structure. These amino acids are often far apart in the polypeptide. The bonding causes this chain to develop specific shapes. Examples are the **alpha helix** and the **beta (pleated) sheet**.

The **tertiary structure** is the three-dimensional folding of the alpha helix or the pleated sheet. Other bonds (e.g., disulfide bridges) between nonadjacent amino acids of a polypeptide produce this level of structure.

The **quaternary structure** is the spatial relationship between the different polypeptides in the protein. The protein part of hemoglobin, for example, consists of four polypeptides. **Insulin**, a hormone that decreases the concentration of glucose in the blood, consists of two polypeptides.

Denaturation is the disruption of protein structure by heating or other means.

1.5 Biological Functions of Proteins

The tremendous variety of protein structures accounts for the wide variety of functions of these molecules. Some of the major biological functions of proteins are:

Structure—They compose the makeup of hair, bones, and muscles. **Keratin**, for example, is a protein found in hair. By shape it is a **fibrous protein** and insoluble in water. **Collagen** is a protein found in ligaments and tendons.

Regulation—Some **hormones** are proteins. Hormones act as chemical messengers transported in the blood. They control body processes. **Insulin,** for example, controls the concentration of glucose in the blood.

Transport—**Hemoglobin** transports oxygen in the blood. By shape it is a **globular protein** and is soluble in water.

Contraction—**Actin** and **myosin** are contractile proteins in muscles. These proteins slide together, shortening the muscle and producing muscle contraction for body movement.

Catalysts—All **enzymes**, which are organic catalysts, are mainly protein. The digestion of starch requires an enzyme. Every step of human **metabolism** requires an enzyme in order to function rapidly enough to support life. Metabolism is the sum of all chemical reactions that occur in the organism.

CHAPTER 2

Enzymes

2.1 Enzyme Structure and Function

2.1.1 Enzyme Action

Enzymes are the **catalysts** for the chemical reactions in living organisms. A catalyst increases the rate of a chemical reaction while remaining unchanged in the process. In order to occur rapidly enough to support life, every step of **metabolism** requires an enzyme.

The structure of an enzyme determines how it functions. Most enzymes are mainly protein. The **apoenzyme** alone is the protein component. How enzymes function in different temperatures and pH environments is related to how proteins react in these settings.

The **cofactor** is the nonprotein part of the enzyme. Often this is an organic molecule called the **coenzyme**, which can be a **vitamin**. In some cases the cofactor is a mineral (metal ion). Without its cofactor, an enzyme is not structurally complete and cannot function as a catalyst. The complete enzyme-cofactor complex is called the **holoenzyme**. Vitamins and minerals are needed in the diet to complete the makeup of enzymes.

The **substrate** is the reactant that an enzyme changes into a **product** in a chemical reaction. An enzyme is **specific** for the substrate it changes. In the following chemical reaction, **catalase** is the enzyme. Hydrogen peroxide (H_2O_2) is the substrate. Water and oxygen are the products.

$$\text{catalase}$$
$$2H_2O_2 \longrightarrow 2H_2O + O_2$$

2.1.2 Enzyme Specificity

Enzyme specificity is related to the **shape** of this molecule. The shape of catalase fits into hydrogen peroxide. However, it is not complementary to another molecule, such as starch. The shape of an enzyme is determined by the **four** different **levels** of **protein structure**.

2.2 Classes of Enzymes

Enzymes are classified by the kinds of reactions they catalyze. There are six major classes. Most of the names of enzymes end in the suffix **-ase**.

2.2.1 Hydrolases

Hydrolysis is the breaking of a chemical bond by the insertion of a water molecule. The chemical digestion of carbohydrates, lipids, and proteins into smaller molecules is an example of hydrolysis. Salivary **amylase** is the hydrolase for digesting starch (polysaccharide) into maltose (disaccharide). Starch is the substrate. Maltose is the product. This chemical change occurs when starch is digested in the oral cavity of the human body.

2.2.2 Isomerases

Isomers are **compounds** (two or more elements combined) with the same **molecular formula** but different **structural formulas**. For example, the sugars glucose and fructose (monosaccharides) have the same molecular formula ($C_6H_{12}O_6$). However, they have different structural formulas (see Figure 2–1). An isomerase is an enzyme that can convert one isomer into another.

2.2.3 Oxidoreductases

Oxidation is the loss of hydrogen (or electrons) from a substrate. **Reduction** is the gain of hydrogen (or electrons). These two kinds of reactions occur together. Often another molecule connects these two kinds

10

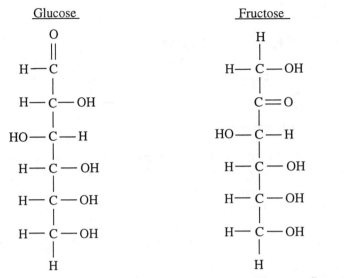

Figure 2–1: Structural Formulas of Glucose and Fructose/Isomers

of reactions. **NAD** (Nicotinamide Adenine Dinucleotide), for example, accepts hydrogen from a substrate during oxidation and delivers hydrogen to another substance during reduction.

2.2.4 Ligases

Ligate means to tie together. A **ligase** bonds two substrate molecules together, building a larger molecule. The molecule **ATP** (adenosine triphosphate) provides energy to build the larger molecule.

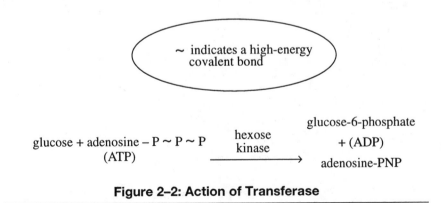

Figure 2–2: Action of Transferase

2.2.5 Lyases

Lysis is a breakage. A **lyase** catalyzes the breakage of a small molecule away from a larger one. Often this reaction is **reversible** and the same lyase catalyzes the attachment of the smaller molecule to the larger molecule.

2.2.6 Transferases

These enzymes transfer a specific group from one molecule to another. For example, **hexose kinase** is a **transferase** that removes the terminal phosphate of ATP. This terminal bond stores high energy. ATP is changed into ADP (adenosine diphosphate). The enzyme transfers this phosphate group to glucose to form glucose-6–phosphate (see Figure 2–2). This is the first step in cells to metabolize glucose for energy.

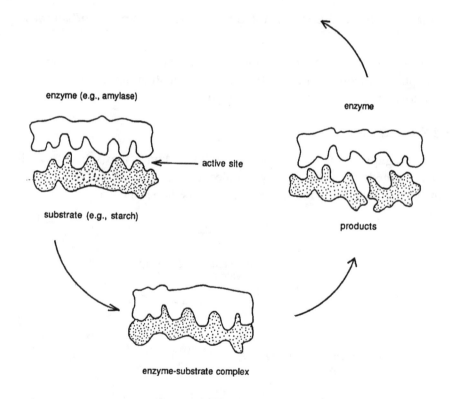

Figure 2–3: Enzyme-Substrate Action

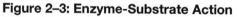

2.3 Mechanism of Enzyme Action

The action of an enzyme is **specific**. The substrate binds to an enzyme at the active site. This site occupies only a small fraction of the total area of the enzyme and is determined by the amino acid sequence of the enzyme. The shape of the active site of the enzyme and substrate are complementary.

2.3.1 Models of Action

The combination of substrate and enzyme is similar to how a key (substrate) fits into a lock (enzyme). Therefore, this interaction was originally called the **lock and key model**. Enzyme **specificity** is related to the complementary shapes of the enzyme and substrate molecules. Each substrate, or key, fits into a specific enzyme, or lock.

The **induced-fit model** is a modern interpretation of the interaction of enzyme and substrate. It recognizes that these molecules are not rigid; they are flexible. As they combine, each molecule induces the proper fit of the other one. An enzyme, for example, can conform to the shape of the substrate. As it does this it places a strain on the chemical bonds in the substrate. This can chemically change the substrate.

2.3.2 Substrate Interactions

When the enzyme and substrate combine, they form an intermediate combination, the **enzyme-substrate complex**. They are attracted by several kinds of bonds, including ionic attractions and hydrogen bonding. This combination forces the substrate into a less stable shape. This breaks some chemical bonds in the substrate and forms new ones. In the process, the substrate molecule is changed into a product.

An enzyme is specific in its action. In Figure 2–3, **amylase** changes the substrate **starch** into **maltose**. This chemical change occurs when starch is digested. After the product is formed and released, the enzyme amylase can combine with another substrate molecule and change it into a product. Starch is a carbohydrate. The digestion of a lipid or protein requires different specific enzymes.

Each enzyme has a **turnover number**, the number of substrate molecules it changes into product per unit of time. For example, its

13

turnover number is 10 if it converts 10 substrate molecules into product per second.

Chemical reactions have an **energy barrier**, or **energy of activation**, that must be overcome in order for the reaction to occur. As a catalyst, an enzyme does not change the energy levels of the substrate and product. However, by inducing a strain on the chemical bonds in the substrate, an enzyme lowers the activation energy barrier. This increases the rate of the reaction. The enzyme acts as a catalyst.

2.4 Factors Affecting Enzyme Activity

Enzymes require certain conditions to function optimally.

2.4.1 Temperature

Enzymatic reactions have an optimum temperature. As the temperature increases, the reaction rate increases to about 37 degrees Celsius. As the temperature continues to increase above 37 degrees, the reaction rate gradually decreases (see Figure 2–4).

As the temperature increases to 37 degrees, the motion of reacting molecules also increases. This increases the reaction rate. However, at higher temperatures, the protein part of the enzyme **denatures**. Therefore, the enzyme is disrupted and loses its activity. Most enzymes lose their catalytic ability at 50 to 60 degrees Celsius.

Internal human body temperature is about 37 degrees Celsius. The enzymes of human metabolism usually function at an optimum around this temperature.

2.4.2 pH

Each enzyme has a unique pH that is optimum. Salivary amylase, for example, functions best at a pH of 7 (neutral) in the oral cavity. Pepsin has optimal activity at a pH of 2 (acid) in the stomach. This enzyme begins the chemical digestion of proteins in the diet. Trypsin works best at a pH of 8 (alkaline) in the small intestine. Its enzymatic activity continues the chemical breakdown of dietary proteins.

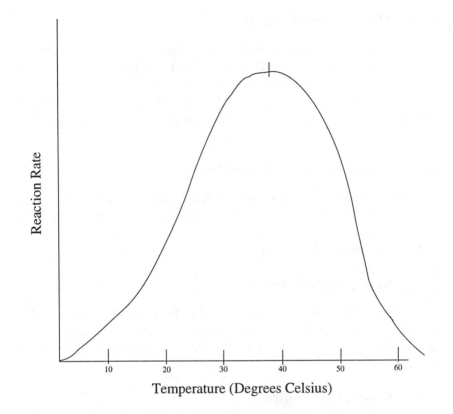

Figure 2–4: Enzyme Activity and Temperature

2.4.3 Enzyme/Substrate Concentration

If the substrate concentration is higher compared to the enzyme concentration, the reaction rate will double each time the enzyme concentration is doubled. This pattern will occur until all of the enzyme molecules are changing the substrate.

If the enzyme concentration is higher compared to the substrate, the reaction rate will increase as the substrate concentration is increased. More and more enzyme molecules will convert the substrate. Eventually, the enzyme will become saturated, a condition in which all of the enzyme molecules are occupied with substrate. Increasing the substrate beyond this saturation point will not increase the reaction rate.

15

2.4.4 Competitive Inhibition

This occurs if a molecule that is structurally similar to a substrate also combines with its specific enzyme at its active site. This similar molecule competes with the substrate for binding to the enzyme. Therefore, less enzyme is available to combine with the substrate to change it. This decreases the reaction rate unless more substrate is added to the reaction.

2.4.5 Noncompetitive Inhibition

This occurs when a molecule that is not similar to a substrate combines with its specific enzyme. This binding changes the shape of the enzyme at its active site and makes it less effective. Its activity is inhibited. Adding more substrate has no effect on the reaction rate.

2.4.6 Irreversible Inhibition

The enzyme forms a strong, unbroken bond with the inhibitor. The inhibitor can be a toxic metal such as lead. The shape of the active site of the enzyme is altered irreversibly. This inhibits the future activity of the enzyme.

2.4.7 Feedback Control

This occurs with a series of steps in a **metabolic pathway**. Each step is catalyzed by an enzyme. In the following pathway the last product, Z, can accumulate and feed back to the first enzyme, E1. It inhibits the activity of this enzyme. This control slows down the additional production of Z.

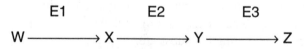

In some cases of feedback control, the last product stimulates the activity of the enzyme at the beginning of the metabolic pathway. This increases product formation.

2.4.8 Allosteric Control

A substance, called a **regulator**, combines with an enzyme and changes its shape. A **positive** regulator increases the activity of the enzyme. A **negative** regulator decreases the activity.

2.5 Vitamins

Vitamins are small, organic molecules that are needed in the diet in trace amounts. The **water-soluble vitamins** (B vitamins and C) are a part of the **coenzyme structure** of enzymes. The **fat-soluble vitamins** (A, D, E, and K) also have important metabolic functions.

Biotin (B vitamin) is a coenzyme involved in the removal of carboxyl groups.

Folic acid (B vitamin) is a coenzyme in amino acid and nucleic acid metabolism.

Niacin (B vitamin) is a part of the coenzyme NAD, which transports hydrogen for oxidation and reduction.

Vitamin B_1 (thiamine) is a coenzyme involved in the removal of carboxyl groups.

Vitamin B_2 (riboflavin) is a part of the coenzyme FAD (Flavin Adenine Dinucleotide), which transports hydrogen for oxidation and reduction.

Vitamin B_6 (pyridoxine) is a coenzyme involved in the metabolism of lipids and amino acids.

Vitamin B_{12} (cobalamin) is a coenzyme involved in the metabolism of nucleic acids.

Vitamin C transports H ions and is an antioxidant.

Vitamin A is a component in making a visual pigment in the rods of the retina of the eye. The rods function in dim light.

Vitamin D is needed for the retention of calcium and phosphorous in the body. These minerals are needed for bone development.

Vitamin E preserves vitamin A and fatty acids. It is an antioxidant.

Vitamin K is needed to make proteins for the clotting of the blood.

CHAPTER 3

Bioenergetics and Cell Structure

3.1 Biochemical Reactions/Energy and Metabolism

3.1.1 Energy

Biomolecules, such as carbohydrates, store energy. Living organisms metabolize these molecules and use this energy to carry out their daily activities.

Energy is the ability to perform work. Energy has a variety of forms. **Potential** energy is stored energy. Water at the top of a dam has potential energy through its position. The energy stored in the chemical bonds of molecules is another type of potential energy. This energy has the potential to perform useful work in an organism.

Energy is neither created nor destroyed. However, it is changed from one form to another. The potential energy of water in a dam is converted to **kinetic** energy, the energy of motion, as it drops in a waterfall. Through **metabolism,** the chemical energy in a glucose molecule is converted into kinetic energy during the contraction of a muscle. During this conversion, some of the chemical energy is also converted into **heat** energy.

3.1.2 Catabolism and Anabolism

There are two major patterns of metabolism for biomolecules. By **catabolism**, larger molecules are chemically changed into smaller molecules. The chemical bonds of these larger molecules are broken, and energy is released. This kind of change occurs when glucose is metabolized and energy is liberated for a muscle contraction or other useful responses by organisms. Catabolic reactions are **exergonic**, since they release energy.

By **anabolism**, smaller molecules are assembled into larger molecules. Amino acids, for example, can be assembled into polypeptides and proteins. The chemical bonds in these larger molecules store energy. Anabolic reactions are **endergonic**, since they store energy.

Catabolic and anabolic reactions are usually coupled in the metabolism carried out by cells. The energy released from catabolism drives the anabolic changes in cells. For example, the catabolism of glucose can provide the energy source to build proteins.

3.2 Cell Structure and Function

There are millions of different species, or kinds of organisms, inhabiting the Earth. However, there are only two kinds of cells that compose these living organisms.

3.2.1 Prokaryotic Cells

Prokaryotic cells are small and have a simple structure. They lack a well-defined nucleus and the membrane-bound **organelles**, or cell parts. A bacterial cell is prokaryotic.

3.2.2 Eukaryotic Cells

Most cells are **eukaryotic**, including the cells of plants and animals. These cells are larger and complex. They have a membrane-bound nucleus and numerous organelles. The organelles are located in the **cytoplasm**, the material between the nucleus and **plasma membrane** (cell membrane). The parts of the cell provide the structures for cell metabolism. Some of the major parts of eukaryotic cells are shown in Figure 3–1.

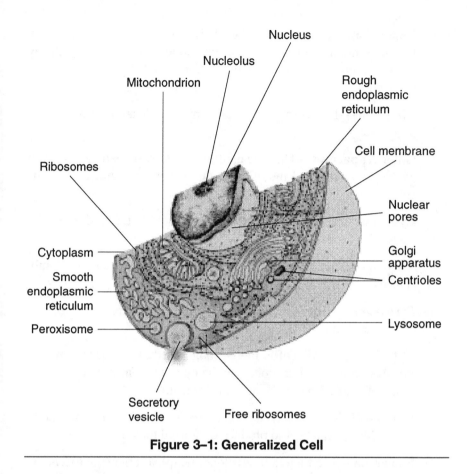

Nucleus

Nucleolus

Mitochondrion

Rough endoplasmic reticulum

Cell membrane

Ribosomes

Nuclear pores

Cytoplasm

Golgi apparatus

Smooth endoplasmic reticulum

Centrioles

Peroxisome

Lysosome

Secretory vesicle

Free ribosomes

Figure 3–1: Generalized Cell

Nucleus—This is defined by a double membrane, the **nuclear envelope**. It contains rod-like structures, the **chromosomes**. They carry **genes**, the units of heredity. The **DNA** of genes encodes genetic information. Chromosomes are visible only during cell division. When the cell is not dividing, the genetic material appears as a mass called **chromatin**.

Nucleolus—This is a spherical body inside the nucleus. It consists of RNA and protein. The nucleoli are made by the chromosomes and compose the ribosomes that participate in protein synthesis.

Centriole—This is a cylinder-shaped organelle near the nuclear envelope. Usually there are two at right angles to each other. The centrioles coordinate the events of cell division.

Endoplasmic Reticulum—The ER is a series of tubular channels. It is continuous with the nuclear envelope. It provides a pathway for the transport of substances. The rough ER is covered with ribosomes. The smooth ER is not covered with ribosomes.

Ribosome—This is the site where amino acids are assembled into proteins.

Golgi Apparatus—This organelle is a series of flattened sacs. It packages, stores, and modifies products that are secreted from the cell.

Lysosome—This organelle stores enzymes that can digest substances.

Vacuole—This is a membrane-enclosed structure that stores substances.

Peroxisome—The peroxisome contains enzymes that catalyze oxidation reactions.

Cytoskeleton—**Microfilaments**, long and thin fibers, and **microtubules**, thin cylinders, compose the cytoskeleton. It maintains the shape of the cell and influences movement.

Cilium—This is a short, hair-like projection of the plasma membrane. Many cilia beat to produce organized movement.

Flagellum—The flagellum is a long, whiplike organelle extending from the plasma membrane. It produces movement for the cell.

Mitochondrion—This is called the powerhouse of the cell. It is usually long and oval-shaped with a double membrane. The inner membrane has folds, or **cristae**, that project into the **matrix**. This divides the matrix into compartments. The matrix and inner membrane contain enzymes and transport molecules for releasing energy from other molecules, such as glucose.

Chloroplast—This organelle contains the green pigment chlorophyll, which can trap sunlight. It is the site of **photosynthesis**. Through this process, the light energy from the sun is converted into the chemical energy of a sugar, such as glucose. The balanced chemical reaction for photosynthesis is:

$$6CO_2 + 6\,H_2O \longrightarrow C_6H_{12}O_6 + 6O_2$$

The chloroplast is found in the cells of photosynthetic organisms, such as green plants.

Cell Wall—Plant cells and bacteria also have a cell wall that is external to their plasma membrane. This rigid covering provides structural support and protection.

3.3 ATP/Energy Transfer

3.3.1 ATP

Biomolecules store energy in their chemical bonds. However, the energy from these molecules usually cannot be employed directly by the cell. The energy from a biomolecule, such as glucose, must be released by catabolic reactions and trapped in the bonds of another molecule, **ATP,** or **adenosine triphosphate**.

ATP is the molecule that the cell spends to provide the energy for its activities. For example, the contraction of a muscle cell requires ATP. The chemical energy from the molecules of carbohydrates, lipids, and proteins is usually transferred to the bonds of one molecule, ATP. ATP is available for the cell. Therefore, ATP is the universal energy currency for cell functions.

The structure of ATP is shown in Figure 3–2. It consists of a nitrogen-containing compound, **adenosine**, plus three **phosphate groups** that are bonded in sequence. The two terminal phosphate groups are connected to the molecule by high-energy bonds. If either of these bonds is broken, a large amount of energy is released.

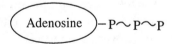

~~~ is a high-energy bond

Figure 3–2: ATP

Often only the terminally bonded phosphate group is broken in ATP to release energy in the cell. The insertion of a water molecule breaks this bond, a process generally called **hydrolysis**. The equation for this reaction is:

$$ATP + H_2O \longrightarrow ADP + P + energy$$

3.3.2 Energy

This is a **catabolic** reaction. Its products are **ADP, adenosine diphosphate**, and the phosphate group. If energy is available to the cell, it can reverse this reaction, combining ADP and phosphate to produce ATP. Cells must also carry out this **anabolic** reaction to restore their available supply of ATP for their functions.

3.4 Metabolic Pathways

3.4.1 Overview

The complete metabolism of biomolecules is not a one-step process. The chemical change of a molecule (e.g., glucose) occurs over a series of steps. This series of related steps is a **metabolic pathway**. Each step is catalyzed by an enzyme.

Figure 3–3 shows the overview of several metabolic pathways. Carbohydrates, lipids, and proteins can be in the diet of an organism. After they are digested into their subunits, they enter cells for additional chemical changes. Glucose, for example, enters cells of the human body for further metabolism.

3.4.2 Glycolysis

Glycolysis is the first stage of metabolism for glucose. This stage is **anaerobic**, meaning that it does not require the presence of molecular oxygen. A series of enzymatic steps converts glucose to **pyruvate**. Some ATP is produced. Pyruvate is converted into **acetyl CoA**. If oxygen is available to the cell, this compound enters the **Krebs cycle** (citric acid cycle). Working with the **electron transport chain**, more ATP is produced.

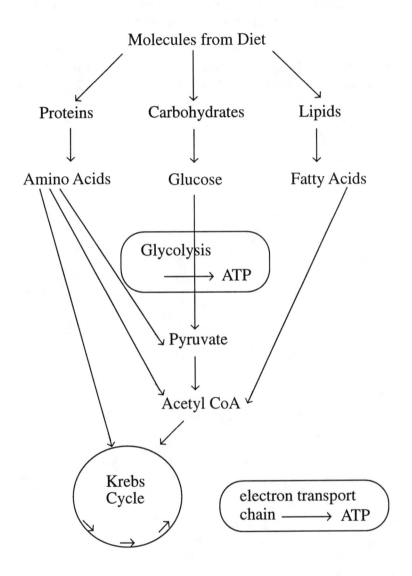

Figure 3–3: Outline of Metabolic Pathways

3.4.3 Krebs Cycle and Electron Transport Chain

The Krebs cycle and electron transport chain are **aerobic** pathways, meaning they depend on the presence of oxygen.

Lipid and protein molecules can also enter at different points in these metabolic pathways for chemical changes. For example, fatty acids and amino acids can be converted into acetyl CoA for ATP production.

CHAPTER 4

Carbohydrates—Structure and Function

4.1 Monosaccharides

Carbohydrate molecules consist of carbon, hydrogen, and oxygen. There are several subfamilies based on molecular size.

Monosaccharides are the building blocks of the larger carbohydrate molecules. The monosaccharides are the simple sugars. They have a sweet taste and a white, crystalline appearance. Most monosaccharide molecules have either five carbon atoms, the **pentoses**, or six carbons, the **hexoses**.

4.1.1 Structure

Important hexose monosaccharides include **glucose** (blood sugar), **fructose**, and **galactose**. These three monosaccharides have the same molecular formula, $C_6H_{12}O_6$, but different structural formulas. Molecules with this relationship are called **structural isomers**. Isomers have different properties. Fructose, for example, has a sweeter taste than glucose.

The structural formulas of glucose, fructose, and galactose are shown in Figure 4–1. These molecules can occur in either the straight-chain form or ring form. Each molecule has a C = O group. When found on a terminal carbon (glucose and galactose), this group is part of an **aldehyde** group. When it is not terminal (fructose), it is called a **ketone** group.

27

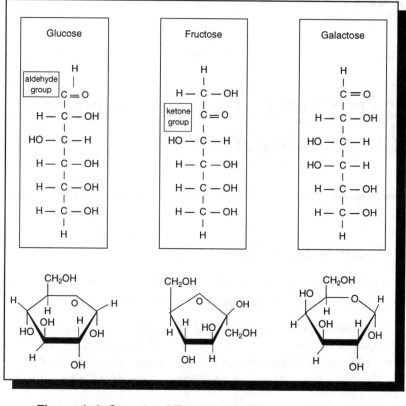

Figure 4–1: Structural Formulas of Monosaccharides

The OH, or **hydroxyl,** groups are bonded to the carbon atoms of these monosaccharides. They are polar and establish positive and negative regions on the sugar molecule. Water is also polar and can dissolve polar molecules. Therefore, simple sugars, such as glucose, are soluble in water. When dissolved in water, the ring form of these sugars is more abundant than the straight-chain form.

4.1.2 Glucose

Glucose is at the crossroads of many metabolic pathways in cells. Often, fructose or galactose is converted into glucose or synthesized from glucose. Lipids or proteins are also converted into glucose or synthesized from this molecule. Glucose is also a subunit for making larger carbohydrates.

The major biological role of monosaccharides is to provide an immediate source of energy for cells. In the human body, glucose is dissolved in the plasma, the liquid part of the blood. When accepted by cells, it is chemically changed to make ATP through the metabolic pathways of glycolysis, the Krebs cycle, and the electron transport chain.

4.2 Disaccharides

4.2.1 Relationship to Monosaccharides

Cells can combine two monosaccharides by a **dehydration synthesis** to produce a larger molecule, the **disaccharide**. By this process, a water molecule is lost between two smaller molecules as they bond together, forming the larger molecule. Important disaccharides are **maltose** (glucose + glucose), **sucrose** (glucose + fructose), and **lactose** (glucose + galactose). Figure 4–2 shows the bonding of two glucose molecules to form maltose.

Another name for the dehydration synthesis is the **condensation reaction**. The formation of a disaccharide from two monosaccharides by this reaction can be summarized by the following equation:

$$C_6H_{12}O_6 + C_6H_{12}O_6 \longrightarrow C_{12}H_{22}O_{11} + H_2O$$

Figure 4–2 shows that one of the monosaccharides loses an H atom and the other one loses an OH group. The H and OH combine to form the water molecule. Each monosaccharide has an unfulfilled bond by its loss. To replace this loss the two monosaccharides bond to each other.

The dehydration synthesis reaction is reversible. A disaccharide can be broken into two monosaccharides by the insertion of a water molecule. This reverse process is called **hydrolysis**. Hydrolysis is chemical digestion. Therefore, maltose in the human diet is normally digested into two glucose molecules. The equation of this reaction is:

$$C_{12}H_{22}O_{11} + H_2O \longrightarrow C_6H_{12}O_6 + C_6H_{12}O_6$$

By hydrolysis, sucrose is digested into glucose and fructose. Lac-

29

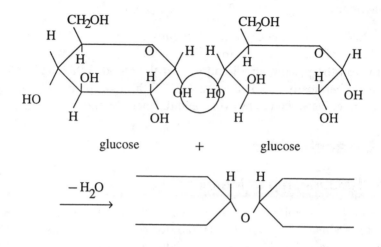

Figure 4–2: Dehydration Synthesis of the Disaccharide Maltose

tose is digested into glucose and galactose. Each hydrolysis reaction in human metabolism requires a specific enzyme.

4.2.2 Function

Disaccharides also provide a source of energy for cells. Maltose is malt sugar. Sucrose is table sugar. It is the major sugar transported by plants. Lactose is a sugar found in milk. After hydrolysis, the monosaccharides of maltose and other disaccharides can be metabolized for ATP formation.

4.3 Polysaccharides

Many monosaccharides can bond into long, chain-like molecules called **polysaccharides**. As cells build into these complex carbohydrates, a dehydration synthesis reaction bonds each monosaccharide to the larger carbohydrate chain.

4.3.1 Starch

Some polysaccharides store energy. **Starch** is the major polysaccharide performing this function in plants. It consists of hundreds of glucose molecules bonded in a chain. There may be some branching in this molecule.

4.3.2 Glycogen

Glycogen is the main polysaccharide storing energy in many animals and the human body. It also consists of many glucose molecules bonded together. Compared to starch, this chain-like molecule has more branching. Storage sites for glycogen in the human body include the liver and skeletal muscles.

Glycogen can be broken into glucose at its storage sites. The glucose is released into the blood, where it serves as an immediate source of energy for cells. This breakdown of glycogen into glucose is called **glycogenolysis**. It is promoted by the hormone **glucagon**. Glucagon is produced by the pancreas.

The pancreas also produces the hormone **insulin**. Insulin promotes the conversion of glucose into glycogen when too much glucose is present in the blood. This process is called **glycogenesis**. When the body stores the maximum amount of glycogen, the extra glucose is converted into lipids for additional energy storage.

4.3.3 Cellulose

Cellulose is a major structural polysaccharide of plants. It composes much of the cell wall in these organisms. Cellulose also consists of glucose molecules bonded together. However, the bonded glucose subunits are aligned differently compared to starch and glycogen.

Humans lack the enzyme necessary for hydrolyzing the bonds connecting glucose in cellulose. Therefore, cellulose cannot be digested by humans if present in their diet. However, cellulose is important as a major component of dietary fiber.

4.3.4 Other Examples

Polysaccharides also contribute structurally to the cell membranes of organisms. They help to anchor other parts of the cell membrane that interact with the environment outside the cell, the extracellular environment.

Polysaccharides can be combined with other molecules to form derivatives. Examples include **glycolipids** and **glycoproteins**. **Chitin** is a polysaccharide derivative found in the skeletons of crustaceans and insects.

4.4 Chemical Digestion and Use of Carbohydrates

In humans, the polysaccharides and disaccharides in the diet are chemically digested. Their monosaccharides can be metabolized for ATP formation. The hydrolysis of **starch** begins in the oral cavity, where the enzyme **salivary amylase** converts this polysaccharide into **maltose**.

The breakdown of carbohydrates in humans is completed in the small intestine of the digestive tract. **Amylase** secreted from the pancreas finishes changing starch into maltose. Maltose and other disaccharides are hydrolyzed into their monosaccharides. Each chemical change requires a specific enzyme. **Maltase** is the enzyme that converts the substrate maltose. **Sucrase** is the catalyst for sucrose. **Lactase** works on lactose.

The monosaccharides produced by chemical digestion are absorbed from the small intestine into the bloodstream. They are transported to the liver for additional metabolism. The blood continually delivers glucose to the cells throughout the body. In some cells, the glucose is converted to glycogen and lipids for energy storage. In many cells, however, glucose is metabolized for ATP formation.

4.5 Metabolism of Glucose

4.5.1 Overview

In most organisms, the metabolism for ATP formation usually begins with glucose or a similar sugar. The balanced reaction for this overall change in glucose is:

$$C_6H_{12}O_6 + 6O_2 \longrightarrow 6CO_2 + 6H_2O + 36 \text{ ATPs}$$

As glucose enters the cytoplasm of the cell, it is first broken down

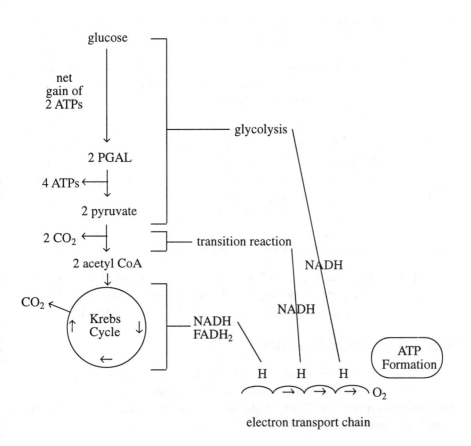

Figure 4–3: Outline of Glucose Metabolism

through the metabolic pathway of **glycolysis**. Figure 4–3 shows the broad outlines of glucose metabolism.

4.5.2 Glycolysis

In glycolysis, each of the steps requires a specific enzyme. These enzymes are located in the cytosol of the cell. Glycolysis is **anaerobic**, as it does not require the presence of molecular oxygen. The key points of glycolysis are:

(1) By a series of enzymatic steps, the six-carbon glucose mol-

ecule is changed into two molecules of **pyruvate**. Each pyruvate has three carbons.

(2) **Phosphorylation**, the addition of a high-energy phosphate group from ATP, occurs in steps 1 and 3. Each step rearranges the atoms in glucose and makes the molecule highly reactive.

(3) After the formation of two **glyceraldehyde 3-phosphate (PGAL)** molecules, two ATP molecules are produced from the further metabolism of each PGAL. The energy for this production is released by oxidizing molecules in the pathway. Therefore, a total of four ATPs are made per glucose molecule. However, there is only a net gain of two ATPs because two ATPs were used in steps 1 and 3.

(4) Two molecules of **NADH** are made per glucose molecule. They remove hydrogens from the metabolic pathway. NADH passes into the electron transport chain to make ATP.

4.5.3 Transition Reaction

Glycolysis is followed by the **transition reaction**. Each pyruvate loses a molecule of **carbon dioxide** and is converted to **acetyl CoA**, a two-carbon compound. This produces two more molecules of NADH, which will enter the electron transport chain.

4.5.4 Krebs Cycle

If sufficient molecular oxygen is available in the cell, acetyl CoA enters the **Krebs cycle**. This is a cyclic series of reactions that occurs along the cristae and inner compartments of the **mitochondrion**. Two turns of this cycle are required to metabolize one glucose molecule, as two molecules of acetyl CoA are produced per glucose molecule.

More **carbon dioxide** is produced by the chemical changes in the Krebs cycle. Most of these chemical changes release energized hydrogens. These hydrogens are transported by the molecules NADH and $FADH_2$.

4.5.5 Electron Transport Chain

NADH and $FADH_2$ pass the hydrogens through a series of acceptors of the **electron transport chain**. These acceptors are embedded in the inner membrane of the mitochondrion. As the energized hydrogens are passed through these acceptors, more ATP is produced. Thirty-two of the 36 ATPs made per glucose molecule are produced through the electron transport chain.

4.5.6 Role of Oxygen

Molecular **oxygen** is the final acceptor in the transport chain, combining with hydrogen to form **water**. Because oxygen is required, the Krebs cycle and transport chain are **aerobic** processes. In the balanced chemical equation for glucose metabolism, oxygen and glucose are the reactants. Water and carbon dioxide are the products. Most of the ATP produced from glucose results from aerobic processes.

If oxygen is not available, pyruvate is metabolized differently. In animal cells, it is converted to a side product, **lactic acid**. In yeast cells, the side product is **ethyl alcohol** and its production is called **fermentation**. These changes do not produce ATP. Therefore the only ATP yield results from glycolysis. If oxygen becomes available, the lactic acid or alcohol is converted back to pyruvic acid for ATP production.

4.6 Photosynthesis

Glucose is produced from **photosynthesis**. This process consists of chemical reactions in two phases: the **light-dependent phase** and the **light-independent phase**.

4.6.1 Light-Dependent Phase

During the light-dependent phase of photosynthesis, the pigment **chlorophyll** traps light energy. This excites electrons in the chlorophyll molecules. These electrons escape and are transferred through a series of acceptors.

The three main outcomes of the light-dependent reactions are:

(1) As the excited electrons are passed through the acceptors, ATP is produced.

(2) Some electrons are passed on to NADP. When an electron and a proton combine with NADP, **NADPH** is formed. It enters the light-independent phase.

(3) Water is one of the reactants of photosynthesis. It undergoes **photolysis**, a breakdown in the presence of light. From this breakdown, oxygen is made. Along with glucose, this gas is the other product of photosynthesis.

4.6.2 Light-Independent Phase

In the light-independent phase, NADPH carries hydrogen to carbon dioxide. Along with water, this gas is the other reactant of photosynthesis. Through a series of reactions, the hydrogens, plus the carbon and oxygen from carbon dioxide, make **PGAL**. PGAL is a three-carbon compound. Every two molecules of PGAL are converted into one molecule of glucose.

CHAPTER 5

Lipids—Structure and Function

5.1 Lipids

Lipids contain the elements carbon, hydrogen, and oxygen. Their molecules contain a smaller proportion of oxygen compared to the carbohydrates. Some lipids may contain additional elements, such as phosphorous and nitrogen.

5.2 Fatty Acids/Triglycerides

5.2.1 Structure

One group of lipids is the **triglycerides**, or neutral fats. The subunits of these molecules are the **fatty acids** and **glycerol**. Figure 5–1 shows each one of these building blocks. Glycerol has a three-carbon chain. Glycerol is an alcohol due to the presence of OH (hydroxyl) groups bonded to these carbons. A fatty acid has the **carboxyl** group, which is acidic. The identity of the R group varies among the different fatty acids, but in most cases is a long hydrocarbon chain.

Figure 5–2 shows a triglyceride. Cells can build this molecule from three fatty acids and a glycerol by **dehydration synthesis** (condensation) reactions. The bonding of each fatty acid to glycerol involves the loss of a water molecule. This process is reversible by **hydrolysis**. Three water

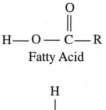

Fatty Acid

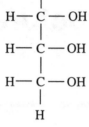

Glycerol

Figure 5–1: Structural Formulas of a Fatty Acid and Glycerol

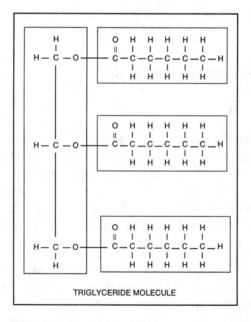

TRIGLYCERIDE MOLECULE

Figure 5–2: Structural Formula of a Triglyceride

molecules can break a triglyceride into its subunits. In humans, this chemical digestion occurs in the small intestine.

Triglycerides are not polar. They are insoluble in water, a polar solvent; however, they do dissolve in nonpolar solvents.

5.2.2 Kinds of Fatty Acids

There are many different kinds of fatty acids. They can differ by the length of the carbon chain of the R group. The chain can range from 4 to 24 carbons, usually with an even number. Some of the most common ones have 16 or 18 carbons. **Oleic acid** and **stearic acid** each have 18 carbons. **Palmitic acid** has 16 carbons.

Fatty acids can be **saturated** or **unsaturated**. Saturated fatty acids have the maximum number of hydrogens covalently bonded to the C chain of the R group. There are no double bonds between the carbon atoms, and all carbons are "saturated" with hydrogens. Figure 5–2 shows a triglyceride formed from fatty acids that are saturated.

An unsaturated fatty acid has at least one double bond between carbons in the R group. This decreases the number of hydrogen atoms that can bond to the carbon chain. Therefore, it is not saturated with hydrogens. It becomes more unsaturated as it has more C-to-C double bonds.

Linoleic acid and **linolenic acid** are unsaturated. They are also **essential fatty acids** for humans, as the human body cannot produce them by metabolism. They must be provided in the diet. Oleic acid is also unsaturated. Stearic acid and palmitic acid are saturated fatty acids.

The triglycerides formed from unsaturated fatty acids are liquids or oils (e.g., vegetable oil) at room temperature. They are commonly found in plants. The triglycerides formed from saturated fatty acids are solids (e.g., animal fat) at room temperature. These triglycerides have more calories because they have more covalent bonds to hydrogen. These bonds release energy when the hydrogens are lost by oxidation.

5.2.3 Biological Functions

Triglycerides store energy efficiently. One gram stores about 9 kilocalories. This is about twice the amount compared to a gram of carbohydrate or protein. Triglycerides also provide insulation and cushioning for the body.

The basic makeup of a triglyceride can be modified to make many derivatives. **Waxes**, for example, consist of long-chain alcohols with fatty acids. They serve as water repellents on plant leaves, animal furs, and bird feathers.

5.3 Phospholipids/The Plasma Membrane

5.3.1 Structure

Phospholipids are another derivative of the triglyceride, or neutral fat. A phosphate group replaces the third bonded fatty acid at one end of the molecule. A nitrogen-containing group can also be present here. The phosphate group tends to lose a hydrogen ion and become negative. The nitrogen group tends to attract a hydrogen ion and become positive. Therefore, this end of the phospholipid tends to be polar and water-soluble.

Figure 5–3 shows the water molecule. Two hydrogen atoms are covalently bonded to the oxygen atom. The shared electrons of these bonds are attracted more to the larger oxygen atom. Therefore, the shared

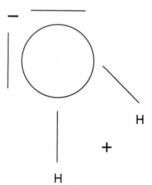

Figure 5–3: The Water Molecule

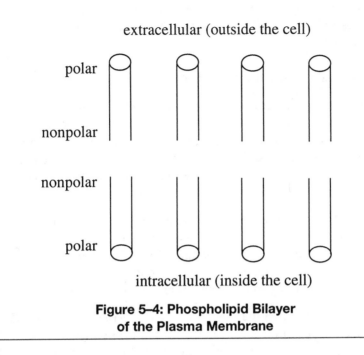

extracellular (outside the cell)

polar

nonpolar

nonpolar

polar

intracellular (inside the cell)

**Figure 5–4: Phospholipid Bilayer
of the Plasma Membrane**

electrons (negative charge) spend more time near oxygen than near the hydrogens. As a result, the oxygen end of water is negative. The end with the hydrogens is more positive. This arrangement makes the molecule polar.

5.3.2 Biological Functions

Phospholipids compose the membranes of cells. For example, the plasma membrane is partly phospholipid. The polar ends of the phospholipid molecules are attracted toward water. The remaining parts of these molecules are nonpolar and are oriented away from water. Cells are usually surrounded by water. Water is the most common substance inside the cell.

Much of the plasma membrane is a **phospholipid bilayer**. Its outline is shown in Figure 5–4. There are two parallel layers of phospholipids. The polar ends (heads) of the phospholipid molecules are **hydrophilic**. They are along the outside and inside of the membrane surfaces, where water is present. The nonpolar ends (tails) are **hydrophobic**. They are directed toward each other at the interior of the membrane, away from the water.

5.3.3 Plasma Membrane Model

Phospholipids are part of the **fluid mosaic model** of the plasma membrane. Other molecules add to the structure of the membrane. Cholesterol is present. Proteins are on both the surface and the interior of the membrane, distributed in a mosaic pattern. The structure of the membrane is not static. It is fluid. The phospholipids and proteins are not anchored, but are constantly changing position.

The changing arrangement of the phospholipids and proteins in the plasma membrane changes its **permeability**. This is the ability of substances to pass through the membrane. There are channels and carrier molecules in the membrane. The arrangement of phospholipids and proteins affects the activity of the channels and carrier molecules.

Transport through the membrane can be passive or active. Gases, such as oxygen, can move through the membrane by **diffusion**. By diffusion, the molecules move from a region of higher concentration to a region of lower concentration. They spread out passively. By **osmosis**, water moves through the membrane by diffusion. Water can pass through the channels in the membrane.

Some molecules and ions move through the membrane by **active transport**. By this process, molecules move from a region of lower concentration to a region of higher concentration. The cell must spend energy for this. The particles of matter are transported by carrier molecules in the membrane.

5.4 Chemical Digestion and Metabolism of Lipids

5.4.1 Digestion

In the human body, enzymes are not present in the oral cavity or stomach to work with lipid substrates.

The digestion of dietary lipids in humans begins in the small intestine. The action of **bile** begins this process. Bile is produced by the liver and stored in the gallbladder. When secreted into the small intestine, this substance promotes the breakdown of large lipid masses into smaller droplets. This is a physical change called **emulsification.**

Next, the small lipid droplets undergo enzymatic action. **Lipase** is the enzyme that catalyzes the hydrolysis of lipids into their subunits. The subunits are absorbed into the bloodstream from the small intestine and are transported to the liver for further metabolism.

5.4.2 Metabolism

The subunits of lipids can enter the same metabolic pathways that change glucose for energy. The liver carries out many of these conversions in the human body. The catabolic reactions of lipids can produce large amounts of energy. Per gram, lipids store about twice as much energy as carbohydrates.

Glycerol can be converted into **glyceraldehyde-3-phosphate (PGAL)**. The glycerol is supplied from the digestion of lipids or the breakdown of stored triglyceride molecules. PGAL enters glycolysis for ATP production. Aerobic metabolism can produce more ATP.

Fatty acids can be converted into **acetyl CoA**. The fatty acids are produced by the breakdown of lipids. In addition, the human body can produce some fatty acids, the nonessential fatty acids, through **lipogenesis**. Acetyl CoA passes into the Krebs cycle and the electron transport chain for ATP production.

Under certain conditions, such as fasting, acetyl CoA is produced too rapidly from fatty acids. Under these conditions, the liver changes acetyl CoA into **ketone bodies**. This change, called **ketosis**, stores energy in these bodies for future use. Some of these bodies are eliminated in the urine. Their production is also recognized by the sweet smell of acetone, a ketone, on the exhaled breath of a person.

Lipids can be synthesized in the body by anabolic reactions. This is an efficient means for storing energy. Acetyl CoA can be used to make fatty acids for this synthesis.

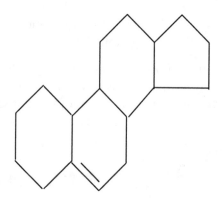

Figure 5–5: Carbon Rings of a Steroid

5.4.3   Relationship to Other Molecules

Glucose and amino acids can be converted into lipids. For example, the hormone insulin stimulates the production of glycogen from glucose. However, it also stimulates the production of lipids from glucose after the storage capacity for carbohydrates has been fulfilled.

5.5 Steroids

5.5.1   Structure

Steroids are not soluble in water. This is a property they share with triglycerides. Steroids consist of a four-ring carbon backbone. These four interlocking rings are shown in Figure 5–5. The bonding of various chemical groups onto this backbone determines the identity of the different steroids.

One of the most common steroids in humans is **cholesterol**. Cholesterol is a part of the plasma membrane. It is also used by cells to produce many other steroid molecules. In addition to its source in the human diet, it is also made by the liver.

5.5.2 LDLs and HDLs

LDLs (low-density lipoproteins) transport cholesterol from the liver to other cells of the body. **HDLs** (high-density lipoproteins) remove this steroid from dying cells throughout the body and return it to the liver. If excess cholesterol is not removed, it is deposited on the inside surfaces of arteries. This can cause blockages in the flow of blood and produce other cardiovascular problems.

5.5.3 Hormones

Some **hormones**, chemical messengers transported by the blood, are steroids. Examples include the **mineralcorticoids**, the **glucocorticoids**, **testosterone**, the **estrogens**, and **progesterone**.

The mineralcorticoids regulate the concentration of minerals (ions) in the body. **Aldosterone** is one example. It signals the kidney to reabsorb sodium, preventing its elimination from the body when it is needed for various functions.

The glucocorticoids regulate glucose metabolism, increasing the concentration of this sugar in the blood. **Cortisol** and **hydrocortisone** are examples. They also reduce the symptoms of inflammation.

Testosterone is one of the **androgens**, the male sex hormones. It stimulates the development of male reproductive characteristics and other male characteristics. Anabolic steroids are very similar to testosterone. They can increase the mass of skeletal muscles in the body.

The estrogens, such as **estradiol**, are female sex hormones. They stimulate the development of many female reproductive characteristics. During the menstrual cycle, these hormones stimulate the development and thickening of the endometrium, the inner lining of the uterus.

Progesterone, a female sex hormone, also stimulates the development of the endometrium. Its concentration and action are high after ovulation. This prepares the endometrium for implantation of the embryo if fertilization occurs.

CHAPTER 6

Protein Digestion and Metabolism

6.1 Chemical Digestion of Proteins

6.1.1 Role of Enzymes

In the human body, enzymes are not present in the oral cavity to work on protein substrates.

The chemical digestion of dietary proteins begins in the stomach. This part of the digestive tract is highly acidic (pH of 1 to 2) from the secretion of **HCl** (hydrochloric acid). This acidity denatures proteins in the diet. The acidic pH also changes **pepsinogen**, which is inactive, into the enzyme **pepsin**. Pepsin catalyzes the hydrolysis of some peptide bonds in the polypeptides of the diet.

From the stomach, the partially digested proteins enter the small intestine. The pH of this part of the digestive tract is basic (pH of 8 to 9). The hydrolysis of proteins is completed in the small intestine. One of the enzymes involved in hydrolysis, **trypsin,** is produced from the inactive **trypsinogen**. **Chymotrypsin** is another enzyme that functions in protein hydrolysis. Many of the enzymes in the small intestine are secreted from the pancreas.

The enzymes that catalyze protein digestion are generally called **proteases**. Each protease works on specific peptide bonds. The **exopeptidases** hydrolyze the peptide bonds of terminal amino acids. Pepsin,

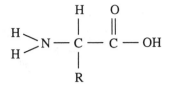

Figure 6–1: Structural Formula of an Amino Acid

trypsin, and chymotrypsin are **endopeptidases**. They hydrolyze peptide bonds that are not terminal.

The hydrolysis of all peptide bonds in dietary proteins produces amino acids (Figure 6–1). These subunits are absorbed into the bloodstream from the small intestine. From there, they are transported to the liver for further metabolism.

6.1.2 Other Molecules

Protein digestion is part of an overall series of chemical changes involving all dietary molecules. If starch is present in the diet, its hydrolysis begins in the oral cavity. Starch hydrolysis is inhibited in the stomach. Salivary amylase does not function in an acidic environment. Protein chemical digestion begins in the stomach. After the action of bile in the small intestine, the hydrolysis of lipids begins here.

The chemical digestion of the carbohydrates, lipids, and proteins is completed in the small intestine.

6.1.3 Nonessential and Essential Amino Acids

There are 20 amino acids necessary for human metabolism. Eleven of these are the **nonessential** amino acids. They can be synthesized by metabolic pathways and are not required in the diet. However, nine of the amino acids are **essential**. Humans cannot make them. They are produced by plants and microorganisms. Humans must obtain these from their diet.

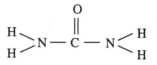

Figure 6–2: Structural Formula of Urea

6.2 Amino Acid Catabolism

The human body has a metabolic pool of amino acids. Some amino acids enter the body from the diet. Others are produced from proteins broken down in cells. Also, cells of the human body can make the nonessential amino acids. The amino acids of the metabolic pool can be broken down by catabolism.

6.2.1 Deamination

Deamination is the initial step in the catabolism of amino acids. This is the removal of the amino group $-NH_2$ from the molecule. The amino group is the nitrogen-containing part of the amino acid. The remaining part of the amino acid can be metabolized for ATP production.

6.2.2 Transamination

By **transamination,** the amino group is transferred to other sites for further metabolism. The amino group can be converted to **ammonia**. The amino group can also be used to make a new amino acid.

Fish eliminate nitrogen from the body in the ammonia molecule. Although this molecule is toxic, it will not harm fish, as they excrete it into the surrounding water. In mammals, however, the ammonia could accumulate in the body. Instead, the liver converts this molecule into **urea** (Figure 6–2). Urea is transported from the liver by the bloodstream. The kidney removes urea from the blood and eliminates it in the urine.

Amino acids pass through the same metabolic pathways that use glucose to produce ATP. After **deamination**, the remaining part of some amino acids is converted into **pyruvic acid**. Others are either converted to **acetyl CoA** or changed into compounds of the Krebs cycle. Therefore, depending where an amino acid enters a metabolic pathway for ATP formation, it can be changed to provide useful energy for cells.

A gram of protein stores about 4 kilocalories. It stores about the same amount of energy as a gram of carbohydrate. It has about one-half the energy value compared to a gram of lipid.

6.2.3 Metabolism

The metabolism of amino acids for ATP production is an example of **gluconeogenesis**. By this process, a substance other than glucose is metabolized for energy. Fatty acids and glycerol can also undergo gluconeogenesis. These other molecules pass through the same metabolic pathways as glucose for ATP production.

In humans, the catabolism of fatty acids, glycerol, and amino acids for energy usually occurs when the glucose is not available for cells. Glycogen, stored in the liver and skeletal muscles, can be broken down into glucose. However, the human body can store only about 400 to 500 grams of glycogen. This can be converted to glucose in less than one day of normal activity.

During prolonged fasting, for example, the body converts all of its stored glycogen into glucose. To continue to produce ATP, the body will usually call on fatty acids and glycerol next. If these molecules become depleted, amino acids are used last. Therefore, there is an order of preference in human catabolism for ATP production: carbohydrates to lipids (glycerol and fatty acids) to proteins (amino acids).

6.3 Biosynthesis of Amino Acids

Humans can synthesize the **nonessential** amino acids. This synthesis requires amino groups. Some are transferred to cells from deamination reactions. Amino groups can also be supplied internally from **glutamate**. This is a molecule that carries ammonia, made from amino acid catabolism, to the liver for urea production. Cells can also make amino groups by other metabolic pathways.

6.3.1 Nonessential Amino Acids

The nonessential amino acids for humans are alanine, arginine, asparagine, aspartic acid, cysteine, glutamic acid, glutamine, glycine, proline, serine, and tyrosine. Although tyrosine is nonessential, it is made from phenylalanine, which is an essential amino acid.

Cells have metabolic pathways to make the nonessential amino acids. One of the precursors for this synthesis is **pyruvate**. Pyruvate is at the crossroads of many metabolic pathways. It is formed from glucose by glycolysis. Some amino acids are also converted to this molecule after deamination.

6.3.2 Essential Amino Acids

The **essential** amino acids for humans are required in the diet. They are histidine, isoleucine, leucine, lysine, methionine, phenylalanine, threonine, tryptophan, and valine.

6.3.3 Role in Metabolism

Humans need a daily intake of protein to supply the essential amino acids. An adult with a body weight of 80 kilograms requires about 64 grams of protein per day. Carbohydrates and triglycerides lack nitrogen. Proteins contain this element. Therefore, the intake of proteins contributes to the **nitrogen balance** of the body.

A **negative** nitrogen balance develops in the body when more nitrogen is excreted than consumed. This can occur when the protein intake is insufficient or a person is fasting. Humans excrete nitrogen mainly in urea. A **positive** nitrogen balance develops when less nitrogen is excreted than consumed. For example, often more nitrogen is consumed in the diet when proteins are needed for the healing of tissues.

Certain foods lack some of the essential amino acids. Legumes (e.g., beans) are low in methionine. Grains and nuts are low in lysine. A diet with beans plus grains and nuts can supply both amino acids. Diets with complementary sources of proteins are necessary to supply all of the essential amino acids.

Many diseases are the result of the lack of proper nutrients or the body's inability to correctly convert these nutrients. **Kwashiorkor,** for example, develops in children from a severe deficiency of protein in the diet. **Phenylketonuria** (PKU) is a metabolic disease resulting from the inability to chemically change phenylalanine. This is due to the absence of the enzyme needed to change it to tyrosine. If phenylalanine remains in the diet, it will increase in the blood. Its high concentration can cause mental retardation in newborn infants. Prevention of PKU requires diets with low amounts of phenylalanine.

6.4 Protein Synthesis

6.4.1 Relationship to Genetics

The assembly of amino acids into polypeptides and proteins occurs at the ribosomes of the cell. The information to make these molecules is encoded in the **DNA** in the nucleus. The **genes** in the nucleus consist of DNA. The flow of genetic information in most cells is as follows: **DNA** makes **RNA** makes **protein.**

The primary structure of a polypeptide is the sequence of its bonded amino acids. With 20 different amino acids, the possibilities for different sequences are endless.

6.4.2 Protein Diversity

On a chemical level, protein diversity accounts for the variety of life forms. Each species contains some proteins that make it unique. These proteins account for its unique structures and functions. This diversity is related to the genetic diversity in the DNA. Each species has specific genes that encode information to make its specialized proteins. There is also genetic variation within a species.

Cells use their genetic blueprint in DNA to program protein synthesis. This strategy has several advantages. Proteins compose the structure of organisms. The human body is about 15% protein. Therefore, genes directly control the makeup of organisms. In humans, bones and muscles contain large amounts of protein.

6.4.3 Enzymes

There is another advantage for the genetic control of protein synthesis. All **enzymes** are made of protein. Enzymes control the steps of metabolism. Therefore, genes also control the metabolism of an organism by programming the enzyme synthesis needed for chemical changes.

Many substances in an organism are protein. If a substance is not a protein, it still requires the necessary enzyme or enzymes for its production.

CHAPTER 7

Nucleic Acids—Structure and Function

7.1 Nucleotides/Nucleic Acids

7.1.1 Nucleotides

Nucleic acids are long molecules consisting of bonded subunits called **nucleotides**. A nucleotide consists of three parts: a five-carbon **sugar** called **deoxyribose**; a **phosphate group**; and a **nitrogen base**. This three-part structure is shown in Figure 7–1. There are two important nucleic acids in biology: **DNA** and **RNA**.

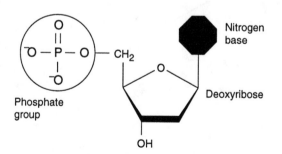

Figure 7–1: Structural Formula of a Nucleotide of DNA

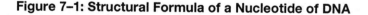

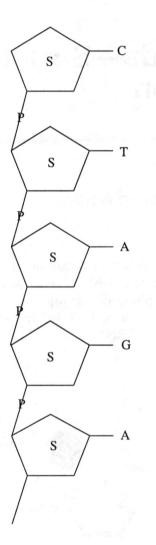

S: 5-carbon sugar
P: phosphate group

Figure 7–2: Single Chain of Bonded DNA Nucleotides

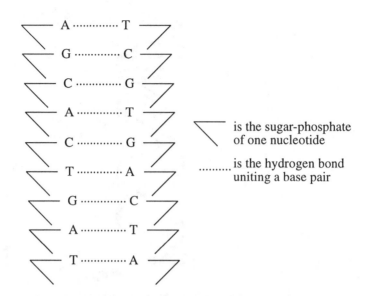

is the sugar-phosphate of one nucleotide

is the hydrogen bond uniting a base pair

Figure 7–3: Double Chain of Bonded DNA Nucleotides

7.1.2 DNA

DNA, deoxyribonucleic acid, consists of two long chains of bonded nucleotides. The base of each nucleotide is either **adenine** (A), **cytosine** (C), **guanine** (G), or **thymine** (T). By these different bases, there are four different DNA nucleotides.

In a single-stranded DNA molecule, many nucleotides are bonded in sequence. The phosphate group of one nucleotide is covalently bonded to the sugar of the next nucleotide in this chain-like molecule. The base of each nucleotide hangs free (Figure 7–2).

The DNA molecule usually consists of two chains bonded to each other. Each chain has a sugar-phosphate backbone. In two dimensions, DNA resembles a ladder (Figure 7–3). The two chains are linked together by hydrogen bonding between opposite base pairs: **A** to **T** or **G** to **C**. The base pairs are the cross-rungs of the ladder. In three dimensions, this ladder-like molecule is twisted into the shape of a **double helix** (Figure 7–4).

55

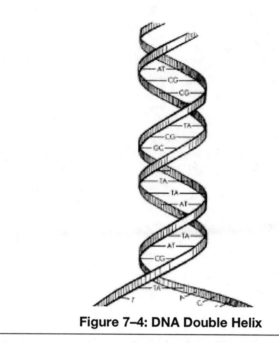

Figure 7–4: DNA Double Helix

The two chains of the DNA double helix are **complementary**. The base sequence of one strand dictates the base sequence of the other strand. For example, if the first seven bases of one strand are ATACGTG, the sequence of the first seven bases in the other strand are TATGCAC. The two sugar-phosphate strands are wrapped around an imaginary cylinder. The base pairs are oriented toward the inside of this cylinder.

One DNA molecule can differ from another by the number, proportion, and sequence of base pairs. The possibilities for different sequences are endless. DNA composes the **genes**, the units of heredity, on the chromosomes of the cell. Therefore, the variety in structure among DNA molecules accounts for the variety in the structure and information of different genes.

DNA is the hereditary material of cells. It determines the development of genetic characteristics.

7.1.3 RNA

RNA, ribonucleic acid, is usually a single-stranded molecule consisting of bonded nucleotides. Each nucleotide has a three-part structure: a five-carbon **sugar** called **ribose**; a **phosphate group**; and a **nitrogen base**.

The base of each nucleotide in RNA is either **adenine** (A), **cytosine** (C), **guanine** (G), or **uracil** (U). The nucleotides are bonded in sequence. The phosphate group of one nucleotide is bonded to the sugar of the next in this chain-like molecule. The base of each nucleotide hangs free.

One RNA molecule differs from another by the number, proportion, and sequence of bonded nucleotides.

RNA differs from DNA in three ways. The nucleotide sugar in RNA is ribose, not deoxyribose. One of the four nucleotide bases is different in RNA, uracil instead of thymine. RNA is usually single-stranded, not double-stranded.

DNA directs the synthesis of RNA in the cell. Through this message, it determines the synthesis of proteins.

7.2 Heredity

DNA composes the **genes** on the **chromosomes** in the nucleus of the cell. The DNA is complexed with proteins, including **histones**, in the chromosome. However, the structure of DNA provides the genetic blueprint for the cell and the organism. Organisms differ from one another by the details of this blueprint.

Genetics is the study of heredity. Heredity is the relationship between genes and the traits they control among parents and their offspring. **Molecular genetics** emphasizes the biochemical makeup of the gene and how it functions.

The **central dogma** states that DNA stores the genetic information to make RNA, which, in turn, makes proteins. This is the order of transfer for genetic information in the cell.

DNA can duplicate its structure through a process called **replica-**

tion. DNA makes RNA through a process called **transcription**. Through **translation** RNA controls the synthesis of proteins.

7.3 DNA Replication

DNA is a molecule that contains the encoded information necessary to duplicate its structure. It does this through **DNA replication.** When a DNA double helix replicates, it produces two double molecules, each with the same number, proportion, and sequence of base pairs.

The process begins when the two chains of the DNA double helix separate. The hydrogen bonds break between the complementary base pairs. Unbonded, the bases of each chain are now free. Each chain serves as a template for the synthesis of a new complementary chain.

7.3.1 Nucleotide Bases

The cell usually maintains a sufficient pool of the four nucleotides to make new DNA chains. Each nucleotide is phosphorylated by ATP to be reactive. The synthesis of DNA is anabolic and requires energy.

The sequence of bases in each separated DNA chain dictates the sequence of bases in the new complementary chain. The **replication fork** is the site where copying begins in the separated helix of DNA. If the first base in either separated DNA chain is A, it will attract a T from the pool of new nucleotides. If the next base is C, it will attract G and so forth.

The base-pairing rules for DNA replication are as follows:

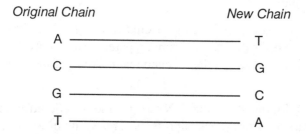

One example is provided in Figure 7–5. If the first nine bases in the free left-hand chain are AGCACTGAT, they will specify a sequence

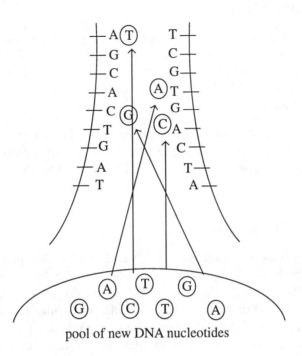

pool of new DNA nucleotides

Figure 7–5: DNA Replication

of bases in the new half that is TCGTGACTA. If the first nine bases in the free right-hand chain are TCGTGACTA, they will specify a sequence of bases in the new half that is AGCACTGAT.

After the nucleotides with bases in each new half are ordered, they bond to each other. An enzyme, **DNA polymerase**, controls this bonding.

7.3.2 Semiconservative Replication

When the replication of the original double helix is completed, two double-chained molecules are produced. Each one is identical to the original double helix. They are also identical to each other. This kind of replication is called **semiconservative**.

7.3.3 Cell Division

When a eukaryotic cell divides by mitosis, the two daughter cells produced receive a copy of each gene in the original cell. For this assortment, DNA replication copies the genes on all of the chromosomes before the cell divides. In humans, there are about 100,000 genes distributed over 46 chromosomes.

In a prokaryotic cell, there is one circular chromosome. The genes on the circular chromosome are copied by DNA replication before the cell divides. Each daughter cell produced receives a chromosome with all of the genes.

7.4 Transcription

Transcription occurs when DNA makes RNA. The process begins when the hydrogen bonds break in DNA and the two chains of the double helix separate. One of the free chains serves as a template to synthesize a strand of RNA, a single-stranded molecule. The cell usually maintains a pool of RNA nucleotides for this synthesis. The sequence of bases in the active DNA chain dictates the sequence of bases in the newly made RNA.

7.4.1 Nucleotide Bases

The base-pairing rules between DNA and RNA for transcription are as follows:

DNA	RNA
A ——————— U
C ——————— G
G ——————— C
T ——————— A

Therefore, if the sequence of the first nine DNA bases transcribed is GGCTACGAT, then the order of RNA bases is CCGAUGCUA. Each RNA nucleotide is phosphorylated by ATP to be reactive. The synthesis of RNA is anabolic and requires energy. After the DNA orders the bases in the RNA, they bond to each other. An enzyme, **RNA polymerase**, controls this bonding.

An **exon** is the active part of DNA transcribing mRNA. A gene is often a series of exons, as their transcribed mRNA molecules are translated into a synthesized protein. The exons are interrupted by **introns**. They are DNA segments that do not code for the synthesized protein.

Some cancer-causing viruses and the AIDS virus reverse the transcription step for the flow of genetic information in the cell. The RNA of these **retroviruses** makes DNA. They have an enzyme, **reverse transcriptase**, to control this process.

7.4.2 Types of RNA

Three types of RNA exist in the cell. **Messenger RNA** (mRNA) is made from chromosomal DNA in the nucleus. It leaves the nucleus and enters the cytoplasm. At the ribosome it provides the genetic instructions to make proteins. **Transfer RNA** (tRNA) is transcribed in the nucleus and enters the cytoplasm for protein synthesis. A tRNA molecule carries an amino acid. **Ribosomal RNA** is transcribed and becomes part of the structure of the ribosome.

7.5 Translation

Translation is the synthesis of a polypeptide from messenger RNA. The sequence of bases of messenger RNA is translated into a sequence of amino acids.

7.5.1 Ribosome

Translation occurs at the ribosome. The bases on the mRNA are decoded in groups of three. These base triplets are called **codons**. The cell normally maintains a pool of amino acids for protein synthesis. Each amino acid is recognized by a specific tRNA molecule. The tRNA brings its amino acid to the ribosome. A base triplet on the tRNA, he **anticodon**, is attracted to a codon of the mRNA.

7.5.2 Nucleotide Bases

The complementary base-pairing rules between mRNA (codon) and tRNA (anticodon) for translation are as follows:

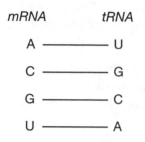

mRNA   *tRNA*

A ——————— U

C ——————— G

G ——————— C

U ——————— A

For example, the codon UUU attracts the anticodon AAA. The tRNA with this anticodon carries the amino acid phenylalanine. Each UUU in the mRNA specifies the placement of this particular amino acid to accurately make part of the polypeptide. The genetic blueprint for this polypeptide originates in the DNA that makes the mRNA.

7.5.3 Three Steps

Overall, translation occurs in three steps: initiation, elongation, and termination.

Initiation—The first codon and anticodon meet at the ribosome. Often, the **start codon** is AUG.

Elongation—The ribosome moves along the mRNA codon by codon, a process called **translocation**. As each codon is translated at the ribosome, another amino acid is properly placed for the polypeptide by its t RNA and anticodon. As more codons are translated, the length of the ordered amino acids increases.

Each amino acid is phosphorylated by ATP to be reactive. The synthesis of a polypeptide is anabolic and requires energy. As the amino acids are ordered, other enzymes form peptide bonds to connect them and form a polypeptide. Additional reactions assemble the polypeptides into an entire protein.

Termination—The synthesis is completed by a **stop codon**: UAA, UGA, or UAG. An enzyme releases the polypeptide from the ribosome. The mRNA is also released from the ribosome.

7.6 Genetic Code/Point Mutations

As a unit of heredity, a **gene** is the DNA that codes for the production of a polypeptide. The function of this polypeptide determines a trait in the organism. For example, a gene in humans codes for a polypeptide in hemoglobin. Hemoglobin is found in the erythrocyte. It combines with oxygen as the red blood cell transports this gas.

7.6.1 Genetic Code

The **genetic code** is a language of 64 codons that specify the amino acids in polypeptides. Four different bases, read in groups of three with repetition, yield 64 combinations. There are 20 different amino acids. Some amino acids have more than one codon. Threonine, for example, has four codons.

7.6.2 Mutation

A **point mutation** is a change in one base of the DNA in a gene. This change can alter the identity of the transcribed RNA and the translated protein. A point mutation can result from an error when DNA is replicating. In addition, **mutagens** (e.g., high levels of radiation) can increase the probability for a mutation.

Sickle cell anemia results from a point mutation. A mutation in one DNA base changes the instructions to place one amino acid in the hemoglobin polypeptide. A different codon is made in mRNA during transcription. This changed codon attracts the amino acid valine instead of the normal one, glutamic acid. The ability of hemoglobin to transport oxygen is reduced.

7.6.3 Human Genome Project

Many human hereditary diseases have been traced to DNA point mutations. The **human genome project** currently is mapping all of the genes on the 46 human chromosomes. A genetic map identifies the genes on a chromosome. The map includes the known mutations of the genes. The genes are mapped in the correct order. The distance between them is also indicated.

CHAPTER 8

Extracellular Fluid/ Homeostasis

8.1 Blood and Interstitial Fluid

8.1.1 Water

Water is the most abundant substance in an organism. The adult human body is about 60% water. It usually contains 30 to 40 liters of this compound. Water is the solvent for a variety of solutes. Glucose is dissolved in the **plasma**, the liquid part of the blood. The plasma is mostly water. Water is a polar solvent. Gases and ionic/polar solutes dissolve in it. Water is also the medium where chemical reactions occur.

8.1.2 ECF and ICF

The water in the human body is distributed through two regions, the **extracellular fluid** (ECF) and **intracellular fluid** (ICF). About two-thirds of body water is extracellular and found outside the cells. About one-third is intracellular, found inside the cells.

A small part of the extracellular fluid (i.e., 25%) is found in the blood plasma. The larger amount of extracellular fluid contributes to the **interstitial** (intercellular) fluid that is found between the cells. Both the blood plasma and interstitial fluid are located outside the cells.

Whole blood consists of several kinds of **cells** and the plasma. The plasma is about 55% of the blood. The plasma is about 90% water. Therefore, the blood is about one-half water.

8.1.3 Blood Plasma

Many substances are dissolved in the plasma, including proteins. The **albumins** are proteins that transport substances and contribute to the osmotic balance in the plasma. The **globulins** (immunoglobulins) protect the body against **antigens** (foreign substances) and invading cells. **Fibrinogen** forms fibrin, a substance that traps cells when the blood clots.

Ions are dissolved in the plasma. Calcium, for example, is necessary for the blood to clot and for muscles to contract. **Gases**—oxygen and carbon dioxide—are dissolved in the plasma.

8.1.4 Blood Cells

There are several kinds of blood cells. **Erythrocytes** (red blood cells) transport oxygen and carbon dioxide. **Leucocytes** (white blood cells) are part of the immune system and provide a line of defense against foreign substances and invading cells. **Thrombocytes** (platelets) initiate the process of blood clotting.

8.1.5 Blood Functions

The blood transports substances. By the pumping action of the heart, it is forced through a series of continuous blood vessels. **Capillaries** are the abundant, microscopic vessels in this transport pathway. At the capillaries, substances leave the blood and enter the cells, meeting their needs of metabolism. For example, oxygen and glucose enter cells. Waste products (e.g., carbon dioxide) move in the other direction.

By its function, the capillary is an **exchange** vessel. Substances move in both directions. They are dissolved in the plasma (see Figure 8–1). As the plasma leaves the capillary it bathes the cells and becomes the interstitial fluid. Therefore, these two parts of the ECF are constantly mixing as they supply the needs of the organism.

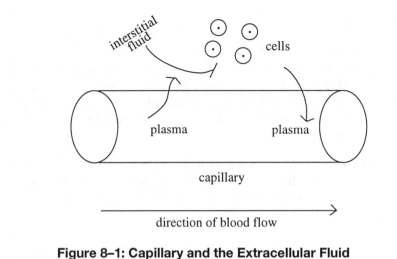

Figure 8–1: Capillary and the Extracellular Fluid

8.2 Homeostasis

Homeostasis is the maintenance of a constant **internal environment**. This internal environment, found inside the organism, is the **extracellular fluid**. The body normally functions to keep the characteristics of this fluid relatively constant. The characteristics of the ECF include **glucose** concentration, **pH**, and internal **body temperature**. To the extent that the body functions homeostatically, it is healthy.

8.2.1 Blood Sugar

The concentration of blood sugar in humans normally ranges from 80 to 120 milligrams per 100 milliliters. The level of glucose in the blood is controlled by at least two hormones secreted from the pancreas. **Insulin**, produced by the **beta cells** of the pancreas, lowers the level of glucose. **Glucagon**, produced by the **alpha cells**, produces the opposite response.

If glucose increases in the plasma after a meal, the secretion of insulin removes the extra sugar. This returns the glucose to a normal concentration. The glucose is taken up by the liver and stored as glycogen. If the glucose level is low, such as during fasting, glucagon stimulates the production of glucose. Its release into the blood returns blood sugar to a normal level.

8.2.2 pH

pH is a scale representing the acidity of an environment. The scale ranges from 0 to 14. A reading of 7 is **neutral**. A reading less than 7 is **acidic**. As the number becomes lower, the environment is more acidic. A number that is greater than 7 indicates a **basic** environment. The pH of the blood in humans is about 7.4. Cells require this pH in the ECF to function optimally.

Acids are compounds that dissociate in water and release hydrogen ions. For example, when HCl (hydrochloric acid) is dissolved in water, it dissociates to produce H^+, hydrogen ions. These free ions are the source of acidity.

Exercise and certain diets can change the acidity in the blood. The blood, however, has substances called **buffers**. Buffers react against the acid or basic conditions of the blood, returning the pH to normal. For example, during **acidosis,** hydrogen ions accumulate in the blood. The buffer **sodium bicarbonate** reacts with these ions, removing them and the source of acidity.

8.2.3 Body Temperature

The average internal temperature of the human body is about 37 degrees Celsius. Water in the blood plasma is an excellent transport medium for heat. Heat travels from a more concentrated to a less concentrated medium. If heat builds up in the body, the blood vessels of the skin dilate. This brings the blood to the body surface where heat can escape. When skin blood vessels constrict, heat is retained.

8.3 Additional Biological Functions

The proteins, carbohydrates, lipids, and nucleic acids are four main classes of biomolecules. Along with water, these molecules perform many functions that are fundamentally important for the survival of the organism.

Some additional functions involving biomolecules are the action of **messenger molecules, fluid balance, ionic balance,** the **inflammatory response,** the **immune responses,** and **blood clotting**. All of these in-

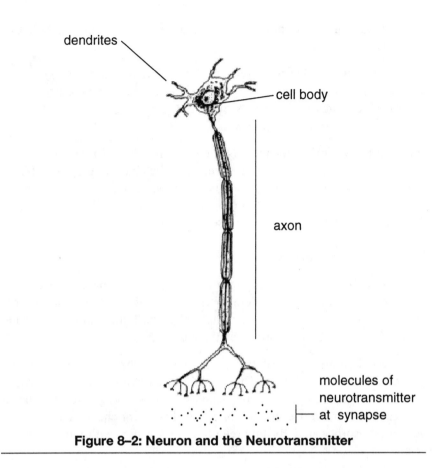

Figure 8–2: Neuron and the Neurotransmitter

volve the blood and ECF. All contribute to body balances and homeostasis.

8.3.1 Messenger Molecules

There are two main categories of messenger molecules: **hormones** and **neurotransmitters**.

A hormone is secreted from an **endocrine gland**. It is released into the bloodstream, traveling to **target tissues** where it has an effect. There are three general types of hormones: polypeptides (e.g., insulin), steroids (e.g., aldosterone), and amino acid products, such as **epinephrine**. This hormone stimulates "fight or flight" responses. For example, it increases the rate of heartbeat.

Neurotransmitters are released from **neurons** (nerve cells). Along a neuron, the signal is electrical. It travels one-way along the nerve cell: from the dendrites to the cell body to the axon (Figure 8–2). The neurotransmitter is stored in the axon.

At the synapse, the signal is chemical. It is a neurotransmitter. The neuron signals the next cell at the **synapse**. The neurotransmitter diffuses across this extracellular space from the axon. For example, skeletal muscle cells are signaled by acetylcholine, a neurotransmitter. Some neurons in the brain communicate by the release of dopamine.

8.3.2 Fluid Balance

Fluid balance in the body results mainly from an intake of water, in beverages and foods, and several outputs. A major output is urine production from the kidney. Every minute, the two human kidneys receive about 20% of the blood pumped by the heart.

The hypothalamus of the brain monitors the **osmolarity** (solute concentration) of the blood. If this solute concentration increases with a water shortage, the hypothalamus signals the posterior pituitary gland to secrete **ADH**, the **antidiuretic hormone**. This hormone signals the kidney to reabsorb water. By this retention, less water is eliminated in the urine.

8.3.3 Ionic Balance

Many hormones regulate the concentration of different ions in the ECF. **Aldosterone**, secreted by the adrenal cortex, signals the kidneys to reabsorb sodium. **Thyrocalcitonin**, secreted by the thyroid gland, lowers the concentration of calcium in the blood. **PTH**, from the parathyroid glands, increases calcium in the blood.

8.3.4 Inflammatory Response

Damaged cells stimulate the inflammatory response. They release substances that serve as chemical messengers. One substance is **histamine**, which dilates blood vessels and increases bloodflow. The blood brings chemicals to repair the damaged area and cells to carry out phago-cytosis (cellular eating).

8.3.5 Immune Responses

Two kinds of lymphocytes, specialized white blood cells, carry out immune responses to protect the body. Several kinds of **T lymphocytes** carry out the **cell-mediated** response. They often react against foreign cells. **B lymphocytes** produce **antibodies**. These molecules, also called immunoglobulins, react against **antigens**. They destroy these foreign molecules.

8.3.6 Blood Clotting

Platelets of the blood swarm to a broken blood vessel. They release a group of **clotting factors** that react in series. The last two substances to react in this series are plasma proteins produced by the liver, **prothrombin** and **fibrinogen**. Prothrombin reacts to form **thrombin**. Thrombin stimulates the conversion of fibrinogen into **fibrin**. Fibrin traps blood cells, forming a clot that plugs the broken vessel.

CHAPTER 9

Glossary of Terms

Acetyl Co: The two-carbon compound derived from glucose (via glycolysis), fatty acids (via beta-oxidation), or amino acids (via deamination), which enters the Krebs cycle.

Acid: Any substance that gives a pH less than 7 when dissolved in water.

Active Transport: The movement of ions and molecules against a concentration gradient, requiring an expenditure of energy.

Amino Acid: The building blocks of peptides and proteins; composed of carbon, hydrogen, oxygen, nitrogen, and sometimes sulfur.

Amphoteric: A substance that is able to act as both an acid and a base.

Anion: A negatively charged ion.

Atom: The smallest part of an element which can combine with other elements.

Atomic Nucleus: Small, dense center of an atom.

Atomic Number: The number of electrons in an atom of an element or the number of protons in the nucleus of that atom.

Atomic Weight: The average weight of an element based on a weighted average of its isotopes.

ATP: Adenosine triphosphate. This high-energy compound is the universal energy currency of the cell.

Base: Any substance that gives a pH greater than 7 when dissolved in water.

Boiling Point: The temperature at which the pressure of vapor escaping from the liquid equals atmospheric pressure.

Buffer: Equilibrium systems that resist changes in acidity and maintain constant pH when acids or bases are added to them.

Carbohydrate: A compound composed of carbon, hydrogen, and oxygen, with the general molecular formula CH_2O.

Carboxylic Acids: Compounds containing the COOH group.

Cation: A positively charged ion.

Cell Membrane: Semipermeable lipid bilayer surrounding a cell.

Chemical Reaction: A process in which at least one bond is either broken or formed.

Chemiosmotic Hypothesis: Peter Mitchell's proposal wherein a proton gradient is established across the inner mitochondrial membrane during electron transport, and the flow of protons down their gradient creates the energy necessary to phosphorylate ADP to form ATP.

Chloroplast: An organelle which is the site of photosynthesis; found only in the cells of plants and certain algae.

Codon: A triplet sequence of nucleotide bases which specifies either an amino acid or a signal to stop translation.

Complementary Base Pairs: The nitrogenous bases of the nucleotides base pair by forming hydrogen bonds according to the following rule: adenine pairs with thymine; guanine pairs with cytosine.

Compound: A combination of elements present in definite proportions by weight and which can be decomposed by chemical means.

Covalent Bond: Bond resulting from the sharing of a pair of electrons between atoms.

Critical Temperature: The temperature at which a substance changes from liquid to vapor or from vapor to liquid and the two are no longer in equilibrium.

Cytochrome Enzymes: The major electron carriers in the respiratory chain, which can exist in either oxidized (Fe^{3+}) or reduced (Fe^{2+}) form.

Cytochrome Oxidase: The last enzyme in the respiratory chain, which reduces oxygen to water.

Dark Reaction (CO_2 fixation): In this second phase of photosynthesis, the hydrogen that results from photolysis reacts with CO_2 to form carbohydrate.

Density: Mass per unit volume.

Deoxyribonucleic Acid (DNA): The molecule comprising chromosomes and genes. DNA is composed of deoxyribose, nitrogenous bases, and phosphate groups.

Diffusion: The process by which a substance, because of its kinetic motion, will spread through or mix with another substance.

Disaccharide: A compound which is a combination of two simple sugar molecules. Examples include sucrose, maltose, and lactose.

Double Bond: The sharing of two pairs of electrons produces a double bond.

Effusion: The process by which a gas moves through a capillary, porous solid, or other small hole in its container into another gaseous region or vacuum.

Electrolyte: Any substance that splits up into ions when placed in solution.

Electron: Negatively charged particle which orbits the nucleus.

Electronegativity: A number that measures the relative strength with which the atoms of the element attract valence electrons in a chemical bond.

Element: A substance which cannot be decomposed into simpler or less complex substances by ordinary chemical means.

Endergonic Reaction: A chemical reaction which requires the addition of free energy.

Endoplasmic Reticulum: An organelle which functions to transport substances within the cell.

Enzyme: Protein catalyst which lowers the amount of activation energy needed for a chemical reaction, thus allowing it to occur more rapidly.

Equilibrium: A situation in which the rate of a forward reaction is equal to that of the backward reaction. There is then no net change in the quantity of either products or reactants.

Exergonic Reaction: A chemical reaction which releases free energy.

Freezing Point: The temperature at which the solid and liquid phases of a substance are in equilibrium.

Gas: A substance in the vapor phase whose atoms or molecules are kept apart by thermal motion.

Glycolysis: The cytoplasmic process whereby glucose is degraded to yield pyruvate, and some ATP is generated.

Golgi Apparatus: An organelle which functions in storage, modification, and packaging of secretory products.

Graham's Law of Effusion and Diffusion: Law which states that the rate at which a gas effuses or diffuses is inversely proportional to the square roots of the gases' respective densities or molecular weights.

Homogeneous: Having uniform composition.

Hydrocarbon: An organic molecule composed solely of carbon and hydrogen, which can exist in chain form or ring form.

Hydrogen Bond: When a hydrogen is bonded to a highly electronegative atom, it will become partially positively-charged and will be attracted to neighboring electron pairs. This situation is termed a hydrogen bond.

Hydrolysis: The splitting of a water molecule into H+ and OH– through interaction with another species in solution.

Insoluble: A compound or other species that cannot dissolve in water or another solvent is considered to be insoluble.

Ion: Atoms or groups of atoms which have lost or gained electrons.

Ionic Bond: Bond created by the transfer of one or more electrons from the valence shell of one atom to the valence shell of another.

Isotope: An atom that has the same number of protons as another atom, but a different number of neutrons.

Kinetics: The study of chemical reaction rates.

Krebs Cycle (Citric Acid Cycle): A series of oxidation-reduction reactions (producing reduced coenzymes NADH and FADH2 which will enter the electron transport chain) and decarboxylation reactions (producing carbon dioxode molecules).

Light Reaction (photolysis): This first step in photosynthesis is the decomposition of water molecules to separate hydrogen and oxygen components.

Lipid: An organic compound composed of carbon, hydrogen, and oxygen that dissolves poorly, if at all, in water.

Lysosome: Membrane-enclosed organelle that functions as storage vesicles for many digestive enzymes.

Meiosis: The process consisting of two successive cell divisions with only one duplication of chromosomes, resulting in daughter cells with a haploid number of chromosomes.

Messenger RNA (mRNA): Carries the genetic information coded for in the DNA to the ribosomes and is responsible for translation of that information into a polypeptide chain. Contains the codon.

Metal: A substance that has the properties of high electrical conductivity, luster, generally high melting points, ductility, and maleability.

Metalloid: A substance having properties intermediate between those of metals and nonmetals.

Mitochondrion: An organelle with a double-membrane; the site of chemical reactions that extract energy from foodstuffs, making it available to the cell.

Mitosis: A form of cell division whereby each of two daughter nuclei receive the same chromosome complement as the parent nucleus.

Molecule: Two or more atoms bonded together.

Monosaccharide: A simple sugar or a carbohydrate which cannot be roken down into a simpler sugar. Examples include glucose, fructose, and galactose.

Mutation: A change in the base sequence of a gene.

NAD: Nicotinamide adenine dinucleotide. This coenzyme functions in many oxidation-reduction reactions.

Neutralization: The reaction of an acid with a base that produces a neutral solution.

Neutron: Particles having no charge that are contained within the nucleus of an atom.

Nucleon: A general term for a particle in a nucleus.

Nucleotide: A complex molecule composed of a nitrogenous base, a five-carbon sugar, and a phosphate group, which functions as the building blocks of nucleic acids.

Nucleus: The dense center of an atom that contains protons and neutrons.

Osmosis: The diffusion of a solvent through a semipermeable membrane into a more concentrated solution.

Oxidation: A reaction in which atoms or ions undergo an increase in oxidation state.

pH: The degree of acidity or alkalinity. $pH = -\log [H+]$.

Photosynthesis: The series of chemical reactions which convert CO_2 and H_2O to glucose and oxygen, in the presence of the energy from sunlight.

Plastids: Structures present only in the cytoplasm of plant cells. An example is the chloroplast which contains the green pigment chlorophyll.

Polysaccharide: A complex compound composed of a large number of glucose units. Examples include glycogen, cellulose, and starch.

Precipitate: An insoluble product of a reaction.

Proton: A positively charged entity that is found in the nucleus of an atom.

Reduction: A reaction in which atoms or ions undergo a decrease in oxidation state.

Replication: The duplication of DNA which occurs in the nucleus of the cell and which precedes mitosis.

Ribosomal RNA (rRNA): Along with ribosomal proteins, it forms an important structural part of the ribosome.

Ribosome: A small organelle which contains ribosomal RNA and functions as the site of protein synthesis.

Salt: An ionic compound made up of a positive ion and a negative ion. Compounds containing the ions $H+$, $OH-$, or $O2-$ are generally not included in this definition.

Soluble: A compound or substance that dissolves in water or another solvent is considered to be soluble.

Solute: A component which is dissolved in a solvent.

Solution: A homogeneous mixture of two or more substances.

Solvent: The liquid into which a solute is dissolved.

Sublimation: The conversion of a solid directly to the gas phase without going through the liquid phase.

Substrate: The molecule upon which an enzyme acts.

Transcription: The synthesis of mRNA based on a DNA template.

Transfer RNA (tRNA): A small RNA molecule for specific amino acids. Carries the appropriate amino acids into the proper positions called for by the mRNA. Contains the anticodon.

Translation: The synthesis of proteins at the ribosome, based on an mRNA template.

Transposable Elements: DNA sequences that appear to move from one part of the genome to another.

Triple Bond: The sharing of three pairs of electrons results in a triple bond.

Valence Electrons: Electrons in the outer shell of an atom.

van der Waals Forces: Weak linkages which occur between electrically neutral molecules or parts of molecules which are very close to each other.

Volatile: The nature of a substance to easily enter the vapor phase.

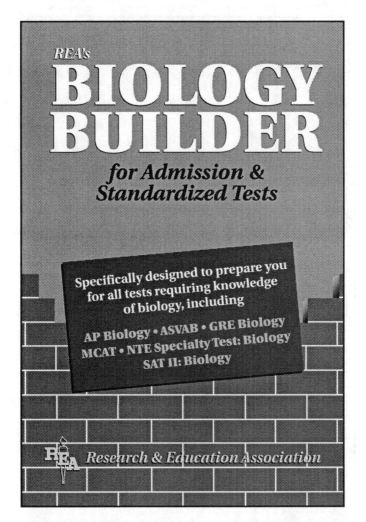

REA's

BIOLOGY BUILDER

for Admission & Standardized Tests

Specifically designed to prepare you for all tests requiring knowledge of biology, including

AP Biology • ASVAB • GRE Biology
MCAT • NTE Specialty Test: Biology
SAT II: Biology

Research & Education Association

Available at your local bookstore or order directly from us by sending in coupon below.

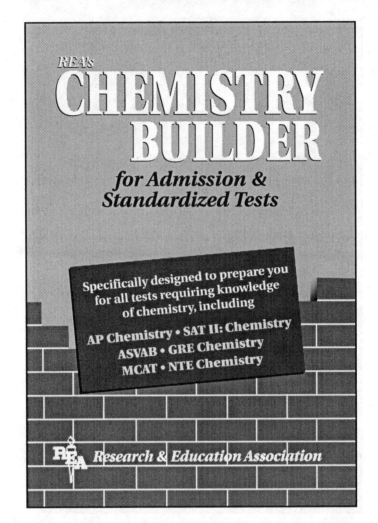

The High School Tutors®

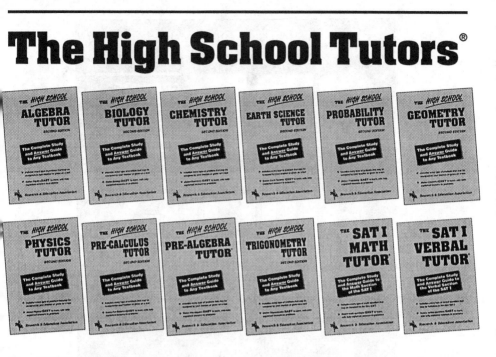

The **HIGH SCHOOL TUTOR** series is based on the same principle as the more comprehensive **PROBLEM SOLVERS**, but is specifically designed to meet the needs of high school students. REA has revised all the books in this series to include expanded review sections and new material. This makes the books even more effective in helping students to cope with these difficult high school subjects.

If you would like more information about any of these books,
complete the coupon below and return it to us or go to your local bookstore.

RESEARCH & EDUCATION ASSOCIATION
61 Ethel Road W. • Piscataway, New Jersey 08854
Phone: (732) 819-8880

Please send me more information about your High School Tutor books.

Name _____

Address _____

City _____ State _____ Zip _____

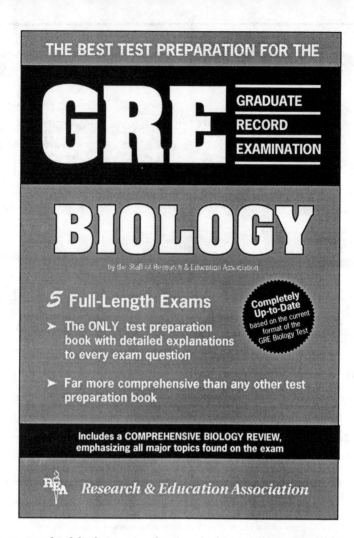

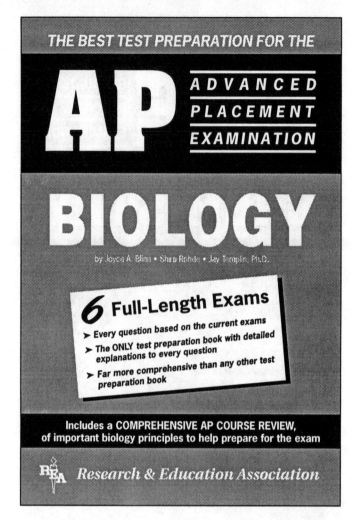

THE BEST TEST PREPARATION FOR THE

AP
ADVANCED PLACEMENT EXAMINATION

BIOLOGY

by Joyce A. Blinn • Shara Rohde • Jay Templin, Ph.D.

6 Full-Length Exams

➤ Every question based on the current exams
➤ The ONLY test preparation book with detailed explanations to every question
➤ Far more comprehensive than any other test preparation book

Includes a COMPREHENSIVE AP COURSE REVIEW,
of important biology principles to help prepare for the exam

REA *Research & Education Association*

Available at your local bookstore or order directly from us by sending in coupon below.